Cuban Health Care

Cuban Health Care

Utopian Dreams, Fragile Future

Mary Helen Spooner and Steven Ullmann

LEXINGTON BOOKS
Lanham • Boulder • New York • London

Published by Lexington Books
An imprint of The Rowman & Littlefield Publishing Group, Inc.
4501 Forbes Boulevard, Suite 200, Lanham, Maryland 20706
www.rowman.com

16 Carlisle Street, London W1D 3BT, United Kingdom

British Library Cataloguing in Publication Information Available

Library of Congress Cataloging-in-Publication Data

Library of Congress Cataloging-in-Publication Data Available

ISBN 978-0-7391-7603-0 (cloth : alk. paper)
ISBN 978-0-7391-7604-7 (electronic)

∞™ The paper used in this publication meets the minimum requirements of American National Standard for Information Sciences Permanence of Paper for Printed Library Materials, ANSI/NISO Z39.48-1992.

Printed in the United States of America

This book is dedicated to our parents and to our spouses, Rhonwyn and Alan, for their love, support, and understanding

"The work that today is entrusted to the Ministry of Health and similar organizations is to provide public health services for the greatest possible number of persons, institute a program of preventive medicine, and orient the public to the performance of hygienic practices."
—Ernesto "Che" Guevara, in a speech to the Cuban militia, August 19, 1960. Obra Revolucionaria, 1960, No. 24.

"At the beginning of the Revolution going to school or receiving free medical treatment for the first time was an incomparable privilege compared with what life was like before. But for today's youth these are established rights for which there are no questions about where they came from or how they are possible. And I am sure that at times when you talk to them about this, they tell you, 'oh, don't come here with the same old speech about health and education.'"
—Cuban foreign minister Felipe Perez Roque, in a speech before the Cuban National Assembly, December 23, 2005, published online by *Granma*, http://granmai.co.cu/documento/espanol05/23dic.html

"Decisions will be adopted in education, public health and the rest of the budgeted sector, aimed at eliminating expenditures which are simply unsustainable, which have been growing year after year and which are not only inefficient but even worse, are undertaken by those who do not feel the need to work."
—Raul Castro, in a speech before the Cuban National Assembly, August 1, 2009, published online, http://www.cubadebate.cu/raul-castro-ruz/2009/08/01/raul-castro-discurso-asamblea-nacional-del-poder-popular/

"Generally, Cuba's medical services are acceptable, although basic medicine and equipment are not always available."
—from the Canadian government's Foreign Affairs and International Trade Department's website section on Cuba, http://travel.gc.ca/destinations/cuba

"Medical facilities in Havana are better than elsewhere in Cuba, but you may need to be medically evacuated if you need specialist care. This can be very expensive. If you need medical treatment you will be expected to pay in hard currency. A basic hospital stay can cost as much as £200 per day plus medical expenses."
—from the British government's foreign travel advice website, https://www.gov.uk/foreign travel-advice/cuba/health

"The hospital's broken windows and screens were an ill omen of worse to come. The black ring (caused by a million grubby hands) around the door handle to the dental ward suggested it hadn't been cleaned since the revolution. We were admitted immediately to the ward and seated at one of a dozen stations. The first image took my breath away. I couldn't believe my eyes. Dental instruments were sitting in a tray that hadn't been cleaned—not even wiped!—in ages. Literally, my best guess is in months, if not years! A microscopic study might well have revealed every known bacteria under the sun. In Europe or North America, the hospital would be instantly closed as a health hazard. The travellers looked up at me with a mix of revulsion and panic."
—From an account of a visit to a hospital in Cienfuegos by Christopher Baker, who led a National Geographic tour to Cuba in 2012, "The Downside of Cuba's Healthcare System," Moon Travel Guides blog, posted January 12, 2012, http://moon.com/2012/01/cubas-healthcare-system-has-its-downside/

Contents

Introduction

When Haiti's devastating earthquake struck in January of 2010, Cuban doctors were the first foreign medical personnel on the scene. Some 380 physicians and other health care professionals were already working in the country as part of Cuba's medical missions abroad and within days dozens more began arriving. A Cuban eye clinic that had been performing cataract surgeries on Haitian patients in downtown Port-au-Prince quickly became a trauma center and field hospital, along with three other Cuban-operated clinics in the capital. The director of the Pan American Health Organization, Mirta Roses, visited one of the clinics and praised the Cubans' work as "excellent and marvellous."[1]

Back in Havana, a very different kind of health care story was circulating. Three days after the Haitian earthquake, the Cuban Health Ministry acknowledged that twenty-six patients at the country's largest psychiatric facility had died from hypothermia and related complications during a cold snap that week. An official communiqué read on state television said that "deficiencies were found in measures taken at the hospital," and that "those primarily responsible for these events will be put on trial."[2]

The Health Ministry's statement came after the independent Cuban Commission on Human Rights reported the deaths, charging that the 2,500-bed hospital had failed to protect those in its care when temperatures dropped.

"The people were not covered up and many windows and doors at the hospital are broken, so they were not protected," Commission president Elizardo Sanchez told the Reuters news agency. "Many of these people are incapacitated and cannot care for themselves." There were "growing signs of deterioration in the national health system," he said, and the deaths might have been prevented if Cuban authorities had allowed international aid groups to tour the psychiatric hospital and the country's other medical facilities.[3]

The Hospital Psiquiatrico Cdte. y Dr. Eduardo Bernabé Ordaz Ducungé bears the name of one of Cuba's doctor-revolutionaries, who took control of the facility a few days after Fidel Castro led his rebel army into Havana. It is still sometimes referred to as the Mazorra Hospital, the surname of the landowner who sold the site to Cuba's colonial authority in the nineteenth century. Cuba's new leaders announced an ambitious overhaul, in which "qualified medical attention was guaranteed and basic needs assured: food, clothing, footwear." Modern psychiatric treatments would be introduced in the context of "respect for mental patients' human dignity as an institutional policy and the introduction of a scientific focus in medical treatment."[4] The hospital began publishing its own medical journal, the *Revista Hospital Psiquiatrico de la Habana*, which still appears three times a year.[5] A baseball team and concert band were organized, and in 1973 Cuba's famed ballerina and choreographer Alicia Alonso introduced a program of dance therapy for patients. The hospital's reform seemed to be a top priority for Cuba's health authorities, and in his report to the first Communist Party Congress in 1975 Fidel Castro commented on the institution's state before the Revolution:

> Under capitalism the National Psychiatric Hospital was a veritable warehouse of sick people, where terrifying scenes occurred and many times the patients died of hunger and mistreatment, to the extent that some directors had a business with undertakers. To say Mazorra was to say Dante's hell.[6]

Accounts of the circumstances in which the twenty-six patients (some dissident groups claimed a higher number) died indicated that sections of the hospital had returned to pre-1959 conditions. Horrifying photographs, purportedly of the victims but impossible to verify, soon appeared on Cuban exile websites and dissident blogs and showed emaciated bodies, suggesting that not only their bedclothes but food rations had been stolen.[7] The case was so egregious that Cuban authorities opened a judicial investigation against the hospital director and some of the staff members, later handing down sentences of five to fifteen years imprisonment. According to the Cuban Commission for Human Rights, the investigation into the deaths did not go far enough.

"It seems that the people who are really responsible will not be tried," Commission president Elizardo Sanchez said. "We were hoping to see the health minister of that time take the blame for what happened."[8]

The Cuban health care system has been the focus of much international attention and debate while revealing jarring contrasts. Long publicized as the Cuban Revolution's greatest accomplishment, it is also a system covered by such a thick wall of political ideology that critical analysis is difficult. Its medical missions in Haiti and other developing countries have generated goodwill toward the Castro government, even as humanitarian groups in North America and Europe organize shipments of medicines and medical equipment to Cuban clinics and hospitals plagued by shortages of the most basic supplies. No country's health care system functions independently of its economy, and over the years Cuba's medical services and public health indicators have improved at some intervals and declined at others, most notably during the early nineties following the collapse of the Soviet Union and the loss of aid and trading privileges that country had provided Cuba. More recently, Cuban authorities have been closing medical facilities and making other cutbacks in the health budget, amid reported outbreaks of cholera and dengue fever in several parts of the country. The Cuban health care system is facing more upheaval as the country begins to look ahead to a post-Castro Cuba and the changes this could entail.

The Cuban health care system is also the subject of American people-to-people tours permitted under U.S. trade sanctions, which prohibit most Americans from traveling to the island without a license. One of the organizations authorized by the U.S. Treasury Department to conduct such tours is Medical Education Cooperation with Cuba (MEDICC), an organization founded in 1997 which works to increase ties between Cuban and American health professionals and more recently received a $5.8 million award from the Atlantic Philanthropies. Since 2002 this group has given MEDICC $16.7 million to "foster exchange with Cuban health professionals, gain insights on Cuba's use of scarce resources to achieve its impressive health outcomes, and promote cooperation leading to better health in Cuba, the USA and poor communities globally."[9] In 2013 MEDICC sponsored eight tours to Cuba and at the time of this writing was organizing a visit for members of the American Public Health Association in January 2014. The cost of the week-long tour, including air travel to and from Miami, a Cuban visa and health insurance, ground transportation, accommodation, breakfasts, meetings with Cuban health professionals, and the services of a MEDICC guide and translator, was listed as $3,500, which seems a rather high price for a non-profit organization to be charging. Participants are offered an insider's view of "one of the world's best-kept secrets—the Cuban healthcare system," with visits to the country's health facilities and meetings with Cuban health professionals.[10]

According to MEDICC, "Cuba's people are healthy, thanks to a universal public health system based on strong community-engaged primary care."[11] Cuba's official health statistics do indicate positive outcomes, with a lower infant mortality rate than that of the United States and a life expectancy of 78.3 years. If every Cuban has access to at least basic medical services—something not enjoyed by most people in developing countries—then one would expect improved health indicators. But a society's public health is affected not only by the provision of medical care, but by such factors as housing, nutrition, sanitation, and physical safety—all areas of obvious concern in Cuba. And with health budget cutbacks, shortages of medicines and other health supplies, the stress caused by such shortages, and outbreaks of dengue fever and cholera, how healthy can Cubans really be?

A pessimistic view is expressed in a U.S. State Department cable, released by Wikileaks, which contains the observations of an unnamed Foreign Service Health Professional (FSHP) at the U.S. Interests Section in Havana:

> After living in Cuba for two and a half years, treating numerous Cuban employees at USINT, and interacting with many other Cubans, the FSHP believes many are malnourished and psychologically stressed. Hypertension, diabetes and asthma are widespread, but poorly treated. Common prescription and basic over-the-counter medications are unavailable. Given the large number of chronic diseases treated by the FSHP, preventive medicine in Cuba is a by-gone ideal, rather than the standard practice of care.[12]

Considering the state of U.S.–Cuban relations, it is hardly surprising that an American official would make such a negative assessment. But a similar view can be found in the work of a Canadian anthropologist, P. Sean Brotherton of Yale University, who researched Cuban health care in the post-Soviet period, and asked a family doctor in southeast Havana how many of the people registered with his practice, or *area de salud*, were actually healthy.

> "Not many," he replied. Between chronic and infectious illnesses, expectant mothers, illegal migrants, smokers, sexually promiscuous youth, alcoholism, criminality and general antisocial behavior, Perez' area de salud was an epidemiological nightmare of risks waiting to unravel into health problems.[13]

Cuba's official health statistics have been challenged by some exile and dissident groups, including former health ministry officials who have left the country. There is no way to independently verify these official figures, which are used by international organizations such as the World Health Organization (WHO) and the United Nations, but there are some anomalies in Cuba's health statistics which will be discussed later in this book.

The authors sought to approach this subject as open-mindedly as possible, seeking the views of a wide range of specialists, health professionals, and the small number of nongovernmental organizations and charities which have been allowed to work in Cuba. Some were helpful and generous with their time, some did not respond to queries and others were extremely cautious. A representative from an American charity for the disabled said the organization did not "want to offer anyone to speak about their outreach in Cuba, for fear of jeopardizing relationships there."[14]

At times, the Cuban security apparatus made its presence felt, even outside of Cuba. One of the authors contacted an academic with many years of experience in the country, who suggested a 2 p.m. meeting on October 22, 2012 at the Salisbury, a pub near the University of London. The author arrived first, found the pub to be almost completely empty, and sat down at a table in the corner. The academic arrived and we began talking about some of his experiences in Cuba, my interest in health care, how the Cuban government responded to requests by foreign researchers, and how best to get around in Havana. After a short time we were interrupted by a child's voice.

"Hola!"

I turned around to see a little blonde-haired girl, two or three years old, sitting at the table directly behind me and waving to my companion. The man with her sat in silence with the back of his chair against the back of my chair, having selected this particular location from the numerous empty tables at the pub. He did not turn around, but stared straight ahead and remained there until we left.

Academic researchers and foreign journalists may or may not gain entry into Cuba and once inside the country are under continuous surveillance and may or may not be allowed access to archives or interviews with relevant sources. Those who do are understandably nervous about losing this access and the effect this would have on their careers or their institutions' Cuban programs, or of getting Cubans who had helped them into trouble. Kathleen Barrett, who went to Cuba to research the effects of the collapse of the Soviet bloc on the country's health care, found her room broken into the day before she left, and that notes, documents, and other materials had been taken.[15] Katherine Hirschfeld, who researched health care in Cuba from 1996–1997, recounts being asked by a Communist Party youth leader to befriend and report on a group of American students in a summer program in Santiago.[16] Foreign delegations visiting Cuba are usually brought to carefully managed locales, with scripted presentations and staged encounters with Cuban citizens expressing pro-government views.[17] Not every tour participant, of course, automatically accepts all that is presented, and there are sometimes opportunities to ask further questions. But many return from these visits expressing favorable views of the Cuban health care system and urging closer ties between the United States and Cuba. The mayor of Akron, Ohio, Don Plusquellic, was one of fifteen members of a week-long trip to Cuba organized by MEDICC in early 2014, at a cost of about $5,000. He later said he was bothered by how the U.S. trade embargo prevented the provision of used medical equipment to Cuba (though in fact medical and agricultural products are allowed) and that he might bring a resolution to the Akron City Council urging the federal government to permit such shipments.[18]

Cuba's own health researchers, working under considerable economic and political constraints, still manage to produce a significant amount of medical literature and the country has over fifty health journals, covering most medical specializations, tropical disease research, and public health issues at the regional and national level. In addition, the Cuban government has collected extensive population data and conducted numerous health surveys at the local and national level. Much of this content is available in libraries or online, and provides at least a partial view of public health issues in the country such as anemia or parasitic infection rates in different communities.

The large quantity of medical publishing within Cuba contrasts with the country's more limited contributions to foreign journals: the representative of the Pan American Health Organization in Cuba, Dr. Jose Luis Di Fabio, has said that Cubans are not publishing enough in international medical publications.[19] And despite the Cuban health system's stated emphasis on primary care, that particular subject is not well covered even in the country's own medical journals.

A survey of five generalist medical journals published in Cuba revealed that less than a third of their contents were dedicated to primary care topics and that many of the articles were written by professionals outside the field. According to Dr. Mikhail Benet, who chairs the Cuban Medical Journals Advisory Committee, there is a great need for more material on the most important health issues facing the country, including Cuba's rapidly ageing population, dementia, increases in obesity and diabetes, dengue fever, and "newly appearing epidemics, such as the recent outbreaks of cholera."[20]

If information on primary care issues is limited, the official news on occurrences of cholera, malaria, and dengue fever is even more restricted, amounting to an "epidemiological silence," in the words of one Cuban physician. Writing in the *Revista Cubana de Salud Publica,* Dr. Luis Suárez Rosas, a professor at the National School of Public Health, recounted previous disease outbreaks in Cuban history, such as yellow fever and newborn tetanus, which were successfully eradicated by public health officials in the early twentieth century. He noted there was no shortage of scientific knowledge or any lack of experience in this area among Cuban health professionals and said that when official acknowledgement of a health threat is lacking, "numerous unofficial rumors circulate," which undermine efforts to control disease.[21] The article was a rare, albeit indirect, critique of Cuban government health policy.

Anthony Redmond, a British physician who has toured health facilities in Havana and some of the country's missions in Haiti, describes a "ruthless pragmatism" in the Cuban health care system, which he says has improved public health for a fraction of the cost of a similar improvement in other countries. "Overall your child is far less likely to die and you are more likely to live much longer than you were a generation ago," he said. "But some individuals with rare or expensive to treat conditions may find their health needs unmet under such a system."[22]

More scathing views of the country's health care system come from Cuban doctors who have left the island, whose detailed accounts of patient neglect, lack of basic medical supplies, and political intimidation can in no way be dismissed as propaganda. All of those consulted by the authors professed pride in Cuba's long medical tradition and criticisms of specific programs, such as the Castro government's medical missions abroad, were tempered with kinder words for some of their colleagues' service and dedication. Dr. Eloy Gonzalez, a Cuban doctor who received political asylum in the United States in 1999 and writes a blog on Cuban health care, described the system as "paradoxical."

Cuba is a country with difficulties in producing and dispensing aspirin, while excellent doctors and researchers develop monoclonal antibodies and other medications in a pretty acceptable biotechnology industry," he said. "Many times there are no supplies for suturing a wound in a country where thousands of kidney transplants have been performed. You can wait too long to receive attention at any level of health while a Cuban doctor or specialist undertakes work with dedication and professionalism in countries as varied as the Pacific Islands or South Africa."[23]

This book aims to examine the state of health care in Cuba and what the system might look like in the future. The first chapter is an overview of the country's medical history, and it should be pointed out that even historians broadly sympathetic to the Castro government admit that prior to the revolution Cuba had one of the better health care provisions in the hemisphere.[24] The authors look at institutional changes before and after the 1959 revolution and the government's handling of some of the diseases prevalent in the tropics—dengue fever, cholera, and in the later part of the twentieth century, HIV/AIDS.

The second chapter looks at the chronic shortages and infrastructure problems in Cuban health care, especially in wake of the collapse of the Soviet Union and the end of aid and preferential trade arrangements. How much real care can a physician provide in the absence of equipment and medicines?

The third chapter examines health issues affecting Cuban women and children. The Cuban birth rate is the lowest in the Americas, and one of the lowest in the world, as women simply choose not to have babies, despite the availability of at least a basic level of prenatal and pediatric care.

The fourth chapter looks at Cuba's elderly, whose share of the country's population is growing as birth rates fall and emigration reduces the number of working age adults to support this group. Fidel and Raul Castro's generation have seen life expectancy increased, but the situation of elderly Cubans is increasingly precarious.

Chapter 5 reviews the long history of medical education in Cuba, its expansion under Castro and its extensive programs for training foreign students, who must pass qualifying exams in their own countries before they can practice medicine.

Chapter 6 looks at Cuba's pharmaceutical sector, its research, and the use of herbal and complementary medicines. The country has an extensive biotechnology sector, which in recent years has suffered from funding cutbacks.

Chapter 7 examines Cuba's medical diplomacy, beginning with its first mission to aid victims of a Chilean earthquake in 1960. Overseas missions which started as purportedly humanitarian assistance have given way to contractual agreements in which other governments pay the Cuban government for medical services.

The last chapter looks at the growing business of health tourism in Cuba, expanded as the country restarted its tourism industry in the 1990s, and what effects restored relations with the United States might have on the health care system. How do Cubans feel about "foreigners' hospitals," such as the facility in eastern Havana where the late Venezuelan president Hugo Chavez received part of his treatment for cancer? And what might health care look like in a post-Castro Cuba?

NOTES

1. Tom Fawthrop, "Cuba's Aid to Haiti Ignored by the Media?" February 16, 2010, Al Jazeera, http://www.aljazeera.com/focus/2010/01/201013195514870782.html.
2. Statement by MINSAP, January 15, 2010.
3. Reuters, "Groups says cold weather killed 24 in Cuba hospital," January 14, 2010.
4. "Reseña Histórica del Hospital Psiquiátrico de la Habana," from the hospital web site http://www.psiquiatricohph.sld.cu/generales/historia.html
5. http://www.revistahph.sld.cu/
6. Ibid. The Mazorra Hospital and other psychiatric facilities were also used to hold political prisoners who were subjected to appalling abuse. See Charles J. Brown and Armando M. Lago, *The Politics of Psychiatry in Revolutionary Cuba* (New Brunswick, NJ: Transaction Publishers, 1991).
7. "Los muertos de Mazorra," posted March 2, 2010 on the blog Penultimos Dias, http://www.penultimosdias.com/2010/03/02/los-muertos-de-mazorra/
8. Reuters, "Cuba tries doctors for mental hospital mass deaths," January 17, 2011.
9. "The Atlantic Philanthropies Award $5.8 million to Medical Education Cooperation with Cuba (MEDICC)," press release posted on MEDICC's website November 12, 2013, http://medicc.org/ns/?page_id=14.
10. From an announcement by the American Public Health Association, sent in an email to the author, August 16, 2013.
11. "About MEDICC," from the organization's website, http://medicc.org/ns/?page_id=27
12. "SUBJECT: CUBAN HEALTHCARE: "AQUI NADA ES FACIL," U.S. State Department cable, dated January 31, 2005, released by Wikileaks.
13. Sean P. Brotherton, *Revolutionary Medicine: Health and the Body in Post Soviet Cuba* (Durham, NC: Duke University Press, 2012), p. 123.
14. Written communication from a representative of Joni and Friends, January 11, 2013. The organization sponsors two trips to Cuba each year as part of its Wheels to the World program to distribute wheelchairs and mobility equipment in developing countries.
15. Kathleen Barratt, "The Collapse of the Soviet Union and the Eastern Bloc: Effects on Cuban Health Care," Cuban Briefing Paper No. 2. Washington, DC: Center for Latin American Studies, Georgetown University.
16. Katherine Hirschfeld, *Health, Politics and Revolution in Cuba Since 1998* (New Brunswick, NJ: Transaction Publishers, 2006), p. 86.
17. An example: one of the authors visited the Convento de Belen center for the elderly in Havana on November 13, 2012, as part a Global Exchange tour of Cuba. Tour members were invited to talk to any of the center's elderly participants seated in an open area of the building. The Cuban woman with whom I spoke answered my questions about her activities at the center, then abruptly changed the subject, averting my gaze and saying she was "very worried about the five heroes," five Cubans con-

victed and imprisoned on espionage charges in the United States whom the Castro government has depicted as antiterrorist heroes. Another tour group member reported a similar exchange with one of the elderly participants.

18. Cheryl Powell and Stephanie Warsmith, "Akron-area officials travel to Cuba to study community health-care practices." *Akron Beacon Journal*, February 25, 2014.

19. Gail Reed, "Interview: PAHO's Presence in Cuban Health: Dr. Jose Luis Di Fabio," *MEDICC Review*, Vol. 14, No. 4 (October 2012).

20. Mikhail Benet, "Cuban Publishing on Primary Health Care: An Inexcusable Absence," *MEDICC Review*, Vol. 15, No 2 (April 2013).

21. Luis Suárez Rosas, "El silencio epidemiológico y la ética de la Salud Pública cubana," *Revista Cubana de Salud Publica*, Vol. 39, No. 3 (2013).

22. Written correspondence from Dr. Anthony Redmond, September 6, 2013.

23. Written correspondence from Dr. Eloy Gonzalez, December 11, 2013. His blog, El Blog de Medicina Cubana is at http://medicinacubana.blogspot.co.uk.

24. For example, Richard Gott, in his book *Cuba: A New History* (New Haven, CT: Yale University Press, 2004), writes that "pre-Revolutionary Cuba was not backward in its provision of medical services. The island had some of the most positive health indices in the Americas, not far behind the United States and Canada" (p. 165).

ONE

Medical Histories

In order to understand the current and future health care system in Cuba, let us begin by stepping back and visiting prerevolutionary Cuba. In some ways the island, roughly the size of Tennessee, has always been ahead of its time, even under Spanish colonial rule. In the early 1800s Dr. Tomas Romay introduced the smallpox vaccine throughout the country and fought a cholera epidemic, becoming Cuba's first public health campaigner. Dr. Nicolas Jose Gutierrez helped found the country's science academy in 1826, introduced the stethoscope and along with Dr. Vicente Antonio de Castro y Bermudez developed the concept of anesthesia.

By the middle of the nineteenth century Cuba was publishing five medical journals.[1] In 1881 another pioneering Cuban physician, Dr. Carlos Finlay, was the first to theorize that yellow fever was transmitted by a mosquito and his work in this area earned him seven Nobel Prize nominations.

In 1937 an institute for tropical medicine and disease research was founded at the University of Havana, focusing on malaria and parasitic diseases. Its founder, Dr. Pedro Kouri, developed new methods for diagnosing and treating these conditions, presenting his findings at international conferences—including his discovery of a new genus of tapeworm, *Inermicapsifer cubensis*—and compiling his research in a four volume textbook, *Lessons on Parasitology and Tropical Medicine*.[2]

By the beginning of the twentieth century Cuba had established a system of social security which provided a free, basic level of medical services such as maternity care and coverage to those who were injured on the job. Beyond this, the government provided partial financing as needed for a private overlay of health care which would later provide a model for health management organizations in the United States. This private overlay was a system of health care cooperatives first started by immigrant groups as mutual aid societies, which would later provide the model for managed care organizations in the United States. At a cost of two to five cents per month, the Mutualist Health Associations provided medical services to its members on an as-needed basis, acting as both insurers as well as providers of care, with oversight carried out by a lay member community board. The Mutualist Health Associations had an obvious incentive to promote preventive care in order to keep costs down, and because members paid whether they used medical services or not, the system enjoyed a steady flow of revenue. The Cuban government began providing some financial support for those who could not afford the cost of the monthly fees, and by 1880 there were at least three hospitals managed by the mutualist societies in Havana as well as several clinics.[3] In 1927 nearly half the population of Havana were covered by these health associations, which expanded to other cities in Cuba and even spread to Florida and other parts of the United States, where they were recreated by Cuban immigrant communities.[4]

Cuba also had a higher than average ratio of physicians to population during the first half of the twentieth century, fluctuating from one doctor per 1,958 people in 1931 to one doctor per 940 people in 1953—a more favorable proportion than in many European countries. Havana had two charity hospitals serving the poor, and while the Cuban capital had a disproportionate share of physicians and medical facilities, there was at least one doctor in each municipality outside the capital who provided health care to Cuba's poor.[5] Cuban hospitals also enjoyed the support of volunteers from civic groups such as the Lyceum and Lawn Tennis Club, a women's society devoted to cultural activities and social service. A 1936 issue of the society's newsletter calls for volunteers to take part in an anti-syphilis campaign—not exactly the kind of activity associated with affluent Cuban women in the prerevolutionary period:

> In connection with the Maternity Hospital, they are trying to organize an anti- syphilis campaign, visiting pregnant patients who for unknown reasons have suspended their treatment. The biggest obstacle is found to be patients changing domicile without advising the hospital. [The hospital] wishes to find a way to provide treatment in different parts of the city, for at present all patients must go to Vedado where the hospital is located.[6]

The island's health facilities expanded under successive Cuban governments, which often made a point of showing them to foreign visitors. In 1955 Drew Pearson, one of the best-known American journalists of his day, visited Cuba at the personal invitation of Fidel Castro's predecessor, Fulgencio Batista. Though Batista is best remembered for his ties to organized crime and Pearson was an outspoken critic of Senator Joseph McCarthy's anti-communist campaign, the Cuban leader managed to impress the American columnist with his social programs. In a letter to a correspondent in Miami, dated November 8, 1955, Pearson wrote, "I don't believe it can be denied that under Batista's rule more schools and hospitals have been built than at any other time in Cuban history."[7] Pearson also wrote directly to Batista after his Cuba visit, stating that he had been "much impressed by the number of schools you have built throughout Cuba and the way you have pushed primary education."[8]

At the same time, the Cuban government did not see its role as the primary provider or financial guarantor of the country's health care system. This changed abruptly after Batista fell and the Castro government came to power. Historians sometimes point to a speech by Ernesto "Che" Guevara to the Cuban militia on August 19, 1960 entitled "On Revolutionary Medicine" as a herald of the transformations to come. In this speech the Argentine former medical student criticized a group of newly graduated Cuban doctors who were reluctant to go to rural areas of the country, asking to be remunerated beforehand, and speculated that had it been a group of *campesinos* who had just graduated from medical school they would have enthusiastically taken up such an assignment.

"They would have requested the most difficult and responsible jobs in order to demonstrate that the years of study they had received had not been given in vain," he said. Guevara predicted that within six or seven years the children of Cuban workers and peasants would receive medical and other professional degrees and spoke of the integration of physicians and other health care workers into the revolutionary movement. Health care services should be provided "for the greatest possible number of persons."[9]

Guevara's speech offered no specifics as to how this would be organized, and the Castro government put him in charge of such areas as industry, the Central Bank and most notoriously, war tribunals and firing squads—but not the health ministry or any other health-related post.[10] The new health minister was an orthopedic specialist, Dr. Julio Martínez Páez, the first Cuban doctor to join the anti-Batista rebels. A black and white photograph taken in 1957 shows Martinez sitting behind Castro and two other rebel leaders in the Sierra Maestra. The other three men are conferring, while the future health minister looks directly at the camera and smiles slightly. He is clean shaven, in contrast to his comrades in arms and his shirt, with epaulettes, is buttoned to the collar.[11]

According to a Cuban government official history, the most prestigious of Cuba's physicians had belonged to the Colegio Medico Nacional, the national medical association, whose members included "doctors with wealthy practices, owners of private clinics, executives of mutualist centers but also very illustrious doctors, scientists and honest and revolutionary individuals who fought clandestinely."[12] When the rebel army took power, doctors from its medical unit and other sympathetic physicians formed their own association, the Partido Medico de la Revolucion, "in order to confront this bourgeois association," which attempted to "continue its hegemony" and "did not recognize that a true Revolution where power would be by the people and for the people had arrived."[13]

Martinez lasted just six months in his post before returning to his previous job as director of an orthopedic hospital, later travelling to Great Britain to study new surgical techniques. He was succeeded by another physician-revolutionary, Dr. José Ramón Machado Ventura, who served as health minister until 1967 and who continued to hold senior posts under both Fidel and Raul Castro. The presence of physicians in the rebel army may have helped to make health care a top issue for the new regime, but this did not result in widespread support from the majority of Cuban health care professionals. Estimates of the proportion of Cuba's 6,000 doctors who left the country in wake of Castro's rise to power range from half to two-thirds, while 750 of the country's 1,000 trained nurses also left.

Cuban authorities began a mass training program to produce more physicians as quickly as possible. Questions arose as to the quality of medical training under such circumstances, but the number of doctors began to recover as the government opened additional medical schools. Recalling the shortage of health care personnel during this period, Fidel Castro told a medical school graduating class in 2005 that 3,000 physicians and a reduced number of medical school professors remained in the country, and that "only a handful" of students graduated as doctors during the early years. The first class of new doctors who had enrolled in medical school, post-1959, graduated on November 14, 1965, he said, and during the first decade a total of 4,907 new physicians were trained in

Cuba.[14] If the number Castro cited is accurate, and one allows for a normal retirement rate of retirement among those doctors who remained in the country, it would mean that Cuba did not recover its pre-1959 physician numbers for at least ten years.

Cuba's new revolutionary doctors were required to pledge their loyalty to the

Revolution and to the "proletariat philosophy of medical science for the good of mankind" and to take a vow against providing medical care in a private setting.[15]

If Cuban doctors had joined the rebel army, the rebel army soon put a military stamp on the provision of health care, mobilizing thousands of citizen volunteers across the country. In 1962 Cuba initiated a national vaccination campaign, with the help of agrarian groups, the Federation of Women and the Committees for the Defense of the Revolution (CDRs). The CDRs were more active in urban than rural areas, but in addition to their role as neighborhood watchdogs on the lookout for any signs of subversion the committees also assisted efforts to control mosquito breeding and contain disease outbreaks.

Newly graduated doctors also had to spend at least one year working in rural communities, even though Cuba's population was at least two-thirds urban and in these same rural areas there were not nearly enough medical facilities in these areas to receive them. But the government began opening clinics and hospitals in the countryside, often making use of existing buildings and or else taking over privately operated facilities, such as the health clinic built by U.S. chocolate manufacturer Milton Hershey for workers at his sugar plant in central Cuba. By 1963 there were 122 rural health centers and 42 rural hospitals.[16]

That same year Havana hosted the Tenth National Medical Congress, attended by around 2,000 physicians. Among the 600 papers presented at the gathering were reports from doctors stationed in rural communities describing how their work formed part of a broader effort alongside literacy programs, land reform and other measures.[17]

The Ministry of Health and Welfare was renamed the Ministry of Public Health, whose Spanish acronym is MINSAP, and charged with coordinating Cuba's expanding public health system as well as the mutualist clinics and private medical practices, which were still allowed to operate for a few years after the Castro government came to power. The revamped public health system's cornerstone was the municipal polyclinic, which offered outpatient services in the areas of internal medicine, pediatrics, gynecology and dentistry. MINSAP provided each polyclinic with extensive written guidelines for health procedures and evaluations, drawn up by panels of specialists from these fields. In addition, the polyclinic health teams were instructed to study and report on "the biological, social and psychological factors that interrelate as determining variables in the health-illness process."[18]

While the polyclinics seemed like a good way of integrating local and national health services, with a focus on prevention rather than cure, both patients and staff were less than satisfied. For many doctors, the polyclinics were a disappointing workplace, often lacking the kind of supplies and equipment to which they had access as medical students. Hospital physicians seemed to enjoy a higher professional status, with better opportunities for career development. Cuba was still reeling from the loss of so many doctors, and the polyclinic health teams were often unfamiliar with the communities they served and the local population's health needs. The new system was functioning as a top-down one, in which a centrally-managed structure provides services based on perceived rather than true demand, with professionals determining the appropriate type and amount of medical services that the population requires.

Demand, on the other hand, involves the perceived need of individuals in the population, adjusted by numerous socio-economic and demographic characteristics. It serves as a richer determinant of care required. The polyclinic teams were supposed to assess their patients' medical data in an integrated way in view of health measures taken, with discussion of these finding by all health professionals and community representatives. But a 1978 study conducted at a well-regarded polyclinic in Havana indicated that the kind of team work and integrated health care envisioned by MINSAP was simply not happening. The polyclinic health professionals tended to present data from their areas of expertise, with no integrated overview and community leaders were not often in attendance during these presentations.[19]

As the health care system now provided free care, moral hazard arose, in which a service or good offered free or at low cost becomes overused or wasted. The overworked polyclinic teams often did not have enough time to undertake preventive or follow-up care. Cuban patients complained of long-waiting times at the polyclinics and of polyclinic physicians failing to refer them to specialists as needed; many opted to bypass the polyclinics altogether and to seek medical care at hospital emergency rooms. Movement from the emergency department to a hospital bed was relatively easy, for while Cuba at that time had a shortage of doctors it still had one of the highest beds to population ratios in Latin America, with 5.5 beds per 1,000 people in 1964.[20] But in these circumstances hospital admissions also meant a lack of continuity of patient care, with each admission being treated as a new medical event, driving up costs and reducing quality.

In 1967 MINSAP took over the last of mutualist health association clinics still operating in Cuba, but physicians and dentists who could prove they had private practices before 1963 were allowed to continue seeing patients privately. Private doctors could write prescriptions to be filled at government pharmacies, but were not permitted to refer patients for laboratory tests.[21]

One of the most significant changes in Cuba's health care system would not happen until 1984, with the creation of the family doctor program, which sought to install resident doctor and nurse teams in every neighborhood in Cuba, with a patient load of around 150 families or households. The doctor and nurse would be housed in apartments above the three-room health facility, which usually consisted of a waiting room, office and examining room. Patients were received from eight a.m. until noon, and in the afternoon the family doctor made house calls. The doctor's office would be open for twelve hours on one Sunday each month, to allow those unable to visit during normal working hours.

According to the *MEDICC Review*, the family doctor program was Cuba's "most daring reform in primary health care," and quickly expanded across the country.[22] But the program was not fully in place for at least a decade, due in part to continuing physician shortages. The Castro government's delay in establishing a family doctor program is curious, given the fact that similar systems had already been in place for a generation or more in most countries with socialized health systems. The family doctor is a patient's first point of contact with the health system, performing examinations and arranging laboratory tests and referrals to specialists as needed while maintaining an overview of the patient's health needs. In many countries patients may choose a family doctor from among a group of physicians practicing at a local medical center. There was no patient choice in Cuba's program, and while the family doctors assigned to specific neighbourhoods had relatively small patient loads and received free housing and utilities they were usually on call 24/7 and covered night shifts at the local polyclinic as well.

Even with the family doctor program in place, Cubans were still using emergency services for health issues that would have been better treated by their family doctors. A study conducted in 1999–2000 by Belgian and Cuban researchers found that nearly 60 percent of visits to emergency rooms in one rural and one urban community involved non-emergency health conditions. Given the fact that family physicians were supposed to be available to their patients at all times, this suggests that Cubans believed that the emergency rooms were more likely to provide needed care than their GPs. The researchers observed that these decisions depended in part "on the patient's confidence in the physician, the perception of his technical capacity, his accessibility and the material conditions he works in." They suggested their findings revealed weaknesses in Cuba's family doctor program and recommended that family doctors be better integrated into the emergency care network.[23]

Family physicians are also charged with monitoring health conditions in their communities, and are sometimes called to account if there is an outbreak of illness or a patient dies unexpectedly. Some family practices have a high turnover of physicians, and postings in more well-to-do neighborhoods are sought after. [24]

Stress is an occupational hazard for health professionals in most countries, and to a lesser extent, burnout—a syndrome of depersonalization, emotional exhaustion and reduced sense of accomplishment. Its prevalence among Cuban doctors and nurses has been the subject of research published in the country's own medical journals, though it is unclear how free Cuban health professionals would feel to report any kind of job dissatisfaction. A 2003 study of 287 doctors and nurses working in primary care and hospitals in Havana reported that 30.3 percent were suffering burnout and 50 percent from symptoms of stress, with the highest levels found among primary care physicians (52.8 percent) and nurses (63.6 percent).[25]

The Cuban health system does not provide for much recourse in cases of malpractice, nor doctor-patient confidentiality. For these reasons Cubans sometimes avoid their assigned primary care facility and seek medical advice from trusted family and friends, especially if their social networks include health care professionals. Katherine Hirschfeld, who studied health care practices in Havana and Santiago in the mid-1990s, reports that when Cubans from her research communities did use the formal health care system, these social networks were still invaluable in ensuring access to scarce medical supplies. Unfortunately, these supplies were often procured on the black market, having been pilfered from warehouses, hospitals and pharmacies.[26]

Hirschfeld also examined early MINSAP documents on health data before and after the revolution and found a number of discrepancies which make it difficult to determine the true extent of improvements in Cuba's public health situation. A MINSAP document published in 1969 reports a rise in polio cases immediately after the fall of the Batista government, which then declined after the mass vaccination program of 1962–1983. Given the exodus of health personnel Cuba suffered and the organizational challenges any abrupt regime change entails, it would seem inevitable that health indicators would show an initial worsening. But later MINSAP documents made no mention of this spike in polio cases. Another MINSAP report published in 1968 lists heart disease and cancer and the two leading causes of death in prerevolutionary Cuba, followed by gastritis and enteritis. Subsequent MINSAP documents listed these last two intestinal ailments as the *leading* cause of death in prerevolutionary Cuba.[27]

It is difficult to gauge how satisfied Cubans have been with their healthcare, though Cuban officials appear to have maintained close monitoring of every medical facility in the country. A report by the Revolutionary Orientation Department's People's Opinion Section collected 10,756 opinions of the services offered at all health centers in the eastern province of Holguin during the second half of 1987 and found that 87.6 percent were negative, an increase of three percent over the previous year.[28] Holguin, it should be pointed out, happens to be the Castro brothers' boyhood home and might have enjoyed a certain amount of additional attention from social welfare and health officials. The report's contents are particularly interesting as the opinions were gathered nearly three decades after the Castro government came to power and its health system would have been fairly consolidated and was not yet suffering the economic consequences from the collapse of the Soviet Union.

The report says that the family doctor program was well-received, but that nearly two-thirds of respondents "point out the deficiencies in several consultation centers." There were complaints that health centers were being built in urban areas, where there were already medical facilities, but not in rural communities, and there were criticisms—some scathing—of medical services in these same urban areas. In the municipality of Gibara, hospital emergency room doctors were often absent or inexperienced. Several patients had died during operations performed by one particular surgeon, including two in a single week, Some health personnel were using ambulances "for pleasure rides and personal business" and several senior citizens were taking advantage of free meals at the local home for the elderly in order to sell their food rations on the side.

In the Calixto Garcia municipality, the local ambulance driver "spends all day at home with the ambulance parked there." The report gathered 118 opinions of the local polyclinic and found that

- Patients arrive at 5:00 am and at 8:00 am are told there are no appointments.
- Of the five doctors working there, four are on vacation.
- Patients are told to arrive at 8 am, though consultations do not actually begin until 9:30.
- Doctors are unable to diagnose some illnesses.
- They give good attention only to their friends.
- A certain doctor "drinks a lot of alcohol."

The Sagua de Tamano municipality had a higher rate of negative feedback than the average for the province, with 96.2 percent of negative opinions, an increase of 15.3 percent over the previous year. Respondents also said authorities should "gather the pigs that roam the urban zones" as a public health measure. The provincial capital of Holguin fared almost as badly, with 91.4 percent negative opinions. The city's Vladimir Ilich Lenin Hospital respondents complained that "the elderly are treated badly," that pregnant women "are left to die in the delivery room," that "most of the operations become infected" and that good attention is given "only to friends and to those who have important positions."

One of the few health issues eliciting a generally positive response in the Holguin survey was the Castro government's AIDS policy, which at the time involved forcibly quarantining patients and which attracted considerable criticism abroad. The report did not mention the number of positive or negative opinions, but noted there was "a high degree of confidence and satisfaction on the part of the population regarding the measures taken by the Cuban Ministry of Public Health to prevent massive contamination; TV programs broadcast to that end are evaluated as good." Respondents suggested that "tests should be made on all women who change sexual partners frequently and on those who go out with foreigners" and that "measures must be taken on homosexuals."[29]

A few years earlier authorities had reacted quickly to the first reports of the disease in other countries, forming a national AIDS commission in 1983 and setting up a reporting system in every hospital to detect any clinical manifestation of the disease. But at the onset Cuba's HIV/AIDS program was marked by secrecy and a certain degree of paranoia. According to Dr. Eloy Gonzalez, who at the time worked as an oncologist at the Hospital Territorial de Cárdenas approximately one hundred miles east of Havana, the first information he and two colleagues received about HIV/AIDS happened when they were summoned to a secretive meeting with the hospital director and the secretary of the Cuban Communist Party. MINSAP officials in Havana appeared to have been aware of the disease for some time, but information was highly compartmentalized and restricted and would not immediately be shared with health professionals at the local level. While HIV/AIDS was making headlines around the world, Cuba's state-controlled media had not reported on the epidemic.

The official told the doctors of an emerging disease affecting hemophiliacs, drug addicts and homosexuals, which "enemies of the Revolution" were attributing to Cuban soldiers returning from Angola. Gonzalez and the other physicians were instructed to keep this information to themselves, while being on the lookout for clinical signs of AIDS—fevers without apparent cause, opportunistic infections, signs of immune system weakness, Kaposi's Sarcoma—while warning that "no one knows if this is a new attack of imperialism." Gonzalez said he was stunned by the Party secretary's presentation and the sparse information it contained about a mortal illness. Cuba's HIV/AIDS program was beginning badly, he said, valuable time was lost and doctors would later realize they had misdiagnosed certain patients.[30]

The first case of the disease was indeed diagnosed in "a heterosexual male returning from duty travel abroad."[31] According to a report by the World Health Organization, MINSAP applied the same epidemiological procedures used to control the spread of other sexually transmitted diseases, testing the sexual partners of those diagnosed with HIV at two six-month intervals after their last contact with the infected individual. The tests were voluntary but the results were released to authorities, and HIV-positive patients had the letters SIDA (the Spanish acronym for AIDS) stamped on their identity cards.[32] This last measure subjected HIV-positive Cubans to considerable discrimination, as identity cards are required for many transactions in the country.

The Castro government opened 14 residential facilities around the country to quarantine patients with HIV/AIDS between 1986 and 1993. The WHO report described the sites as being "like suburban communities on several acres of land with modern one and two-story apartment duplexes that are surrounded by lush vegetation and a small garden. In each apartment lived two persons, who could be friends or couples. Medical care was provided by family physicians taking care of the residents."[33] The patients were effectively prisoners at the sanatoria, and the quarantine evoked memories of the Castro government's forced labor camps for homosexuals in the early 1960s. The sanatoria for HIV/AIDS patients, however, were nothing like the labor camps and the accommodations were probably more comfortable and the food better than what they what many patients had at home. The fact that a visible number of HIV/AIDS sufferers were not from marginalized groups, such as homosexuals or prostitutes, but returning military veterans and other *internationalistas*—doctors, nurses, engineers and teachers—may have elicited a more sympathetic response from Cuban authorities. The Africa connection resulted in 21 different strains of the disease manifesting themselves in Cuba, including 11 strains unique to Cuba which some researchers suspect were the result of "inter-sanitarium sex."

After 1987 testing was expanded to include all patients with sexually transmitted diseases, blood donors, pregnant women, prisoners, army recruits and "those who had travelled to areas with high endemicity of infectious tropical disease since 1975 or who had frequent contacts with foreigners."[34] This last category included those Cubans working in the country's expanding sex tourism industry. Other Cubans who came forward and asked to be tested could be tested confidentially.

The policy of quarantining HIV/AIDs patients may have prevented the disease from spreading to the general population, but it was also expensive and after a time, officials realized, medically unnecessary. At the end of 1993 patients were allowed to leave the sanatoria and receive treatment on an outpatient basis, and ten years later only 40 percent were opting to remain in the sanatoria. By 2012 only three of the fourteen facilities for HIV/AIDS patients were still operating. The official figure for Cuba's infection rate is 0.1 percent, one of the lowest in the world.

Cuban officials' responses to outbreaks of other diseases have followed a similar pattern of secrecy and paranoia, followed by aggressive public health measures. Dengue fever is endemic to the Caribbean, and is caused by a virus carried by the *Ae aegypti* mosquito. Symptoms include headache, fever, muscle and joint pain and a skin rash similar to that of measles. A smaller proportion of sufferers develop the life-threatening dengue hemorrhagic fever or dengue shock syndrome, when blood pressure drops to dangerously low levels.

The disease was first reported in Cuba in 1828, as part of an epidemic that spread through the Caribbean and Gulf regions. In 1850 there was another outbreak reported in Cuba and the southern United States. The disease continued to make sporadic appearances, despite attempts by the Pan American Health Organization to control the vector. [35] In 1981 Cuba suffered another outbreak of dengue fever, with 344,203 people affected and 158 deaths.[36] On July 26 of that year Fidel Castro, speaking on the anniversary of his rebels' failed attack on the Moncada army barracks, said he suspected the United States might be responsible for the epidemic, as well as a recent outbreak of crop disease. [37]

An intensive campaign to control the disease then followed, and Cuban officials later declared the country to be free of the dengue-carrying mosquito species. Then in 1996 the relief organization Médecins sans Frontiéres (MSF) received a confidential request from Cuban officials for 180 tons of insecticide and spraying equipment to kill another variety of mosquito, *Ae albopictus*. According to the British medical journal The Lancet, the request seemed unusual, for *Ae albopictus* is more difficult to eradicate that *Ae aegypti* and its role in the spread of dengue fever is not clear. MSF delayed sending the shipment, then was told Cuba had been using its own insecticide to control *Ae albopictus* and needed additional supplies to complete the eradication program. MSF send the shipment, but denied Cuba a second request for insecticide.[38]

Katherine Hirschfeld arrived in Cuba to research its health care system in late 1996, shortly before the dengue fever outbreak in the eastern part of the country. None of the physicians she consulted acknowledged the outbreak and officials repeatedly insisted that Cuba had eradicated dengue. While working in Santiago Hirschfeld fell ill with the tell-tale symptoms of the disease and was taken against her will to a crowded hospital ward, where she learned there had been thousands of cases of dengue and dengue hemorrhagic fever in the area. She later wrote that during her time as a patient at the hospital, "No physician ever spoke to me about my condition, mosquitoes swarmed throughout the wards, and (other than a single vitamin tablet) I was given no medications to alleviate my suffering. Nursing care was scarce, and ambulatory (patients such as myself) took care of those too weak to move. Since the epidemic was considered a state secret, an armed solider guarded the entry to the ward. I was not allowed to telephone anyone in the United States about my condition."[39]

Cuban sources later told *The Lancet* that the dengue-carrying *Ae aegypti* mosquito had spread rapidly from eastern Cuba from 1992, and that the Pan American Health Organization, which normally monitors disease outbreaks, in the Americas, was unaware of the situation.[40]

A Cuban physician broke the news of the dengue outbreak to the foreign press, reporting over 10,000 cases and 30 deaths. Dr. Dessy Mendoza was then arrested and charged with "enemy propaganda" and sentenced to eight years in prison and released after international pressure a year later, along with another political prisoner. But Mendoza's revelation forced Cuban authorities to publicly acknowledge the outbreak of the disease and mobilized citizen brigades to canvas their neighborhoods for any possible cases of dengue and to take measures to prevent mosquitoes from breeding. Hirschfeld described the anti-mosquito campaign as impressive, with planes spraying insecticide overhead and "men with high-tech motorized sprayers appeared at the door three times in one week to fumigate the house and the patio."[41]

There have been sporadic reports of dengue in Cuba since then, often reported by independent journalists and bloggers. At the end of 2013 an official in the province of Villa Clara told a local radio station that there were700 confirmed cases of dengue in Santa Clara, the capital, along with over a thousand suspected cases.[42] Another hard to control disease, cholera, reappeared in the country in 2012, likely brought back by Cuban medical personnel and other volunteers working in Haiti. According to the Pan American Health Association, there were 678 confirmed cases of cholera, including three deaths from mid-2012 to August 2013.[43]

Periodic water shortages lead Cubans to store water in bathtubs and other containers, which can provide breeding grounds for mosquitoes, while a lack of water facilitates the spread of diseases like cholera. Government health programs can be undermined by sewage, water and infrastructure deficiencies, and this will be discussed in the next chapter.

NOTES

1. José Antonio López Espinosa, "Revistas Medicas Surgidas en Cuba durante la Sexta Decada del Siglo XIX," *Revista Cubana de Salud Publica* Vol. 26, No. 1 (2000).
2. Annmarie Christensen, "Cuba's Jewel of Tropical Medicine," *Perspectives in Health Magazine, The Magazine of the Pan American Health Organization* Vol. 8, No. 2 (2003).
3. Ross Danielson, *Cuban Medicine* (New Brunswick, NJ: Transaction Books, 1979), p. 77.
4. Sergio Diaz-Briquets, *The Health Revolution in Cuba* (Austin: University of Texas Press, 1983), pp. 50–51.
5. Ibid., p. 50.
6. From a notice printed in *Lyceum, Lyceum and Lawn Tennis Club Official Newsletter,* Vol. 14, September–December 1936.
7. From a letter to George Gaston, found in the Drew Pearson papers in the LBJ Library in Austin, Texas.
8. From a letter written to Batista by Pearson dated November 26, 1955, from the Drew Pearson papers in the LBJ Library in Austin, Texas.
9. Ernesto Guevara de la Serna, "On Revolutionary Medicine," from *Obra Revolucionaria* No. 24 (1960). http://www.marxists.org/archive/guevara/1960/08/19.htm
10. Guevara entered the University of Buenos Aires medical school in 1947 but his studies were interrupted by his famous motorcycle trip around Latin America which began in January of 1952. According to sympathetic biographies, such as Jon Lee Anderson's *Che Guevara: A Revolutionary Life,* Guevara returned to medical school in October and managed to complete all remaining course work and pass a final exam the following spring. But there is no primary source material showing that he actually received a medical degree from the University of Buenos Aires, and these same biographies indicate he never completed the required internship but left the country in July of 1953.
11. Biographical data from Cuban government website, http://www.ecured.cu/index.php/Julio_Martínez_Páez and photograph from the Cuban Council of State Office of Historical Affairs.
12. Ibid.
13. Ibid.
14. Speech given by Fidel Castro at the first graduation of students from the Latin American School of Medicine. Karl Marx Theatre, August 20, 2005. Published online at http://granma.cu/documento/ingles05/20agosto.htm
15. A. M. De Gordon, "Health and Health Care in Cuba: The Transition from Socialism to the Future," 2003. Unpublished manuscript.
16. Danielson, op cit., p. 133.
17. Ibid., p. 134
18. Julie Feinsilver, *Healing the Masses: Cuban Health Politics at Home and Abroad* (Berkeley: University of California Press, 1993), p. 39.
19. Ibid., p. 39
20. De Gordon, op cit.
21. Vanessa Bauzá, "Rare private doctors fill medical gaps," *Sun-Sentinel,* January 23, 2005.
22. Connor Gorry, "Primary Care Forward: Raising the Profile of Cuba's Nursing Profession," *MEDICC Review,* Vol. 15, No. 2 (April 2013).

23. Pol De Vos, Veerle Vanlerberghe, Armando Rodrıguez, Rene Garcia, Mariano Bonet, and Patrick Van der Stuyft "Uses of First Line Emergency Services in Cuba," *Health Policy* 85 (2008), pp. 94–104.
24. P. Sean Brotherton, *Revolutionary Medicine: Health and the Body in Post Soviet Cuba* (Durham, NC: Duke University Press, 2012), p. 100.
25. Jorge Román Hernández, "Estrés y Burnout en Profesionales de la Salud de los Niveles Primario y Secundario de Atencion," *Revista Cubana de Salud Publica* Vol. 29, No. 2 (2003).
26. Katherine Hirschfeld, *Health, Politics and Revolution in Cuba Since 1898* (New Brunswick, NJ: Transaction Publishers, 2006), p. 221.
27. Hirschfeld, op. cit., pp. 210–213.
28. Equipo de Opinion del Pueblo, DOP PPC Provincia Holguin, 1988. This report was smuggled out of Cuba and a copy given to the Cuban-American Foundation, which distributed it with an English translation, leading to speculation that the report might be a forgery. Julie Feinsilver, author of *Healing the Masses: Cuban Health Politics at Home and Abroad*, believes it is genuine, as did two Cuban physicians consulted by the authors, including a doctor who had worked in Holguin during the period in question.
29. Ibid.
30. Eloy A. Gonzalez, "El SIDA en Cuba: Del silencio a la verdad científica," *Cubanet*, January 21, 2006, http://www.cubanet.org/CNews/y06/jan06/27o6.htm and written correspondence with the author.
31. World Health Organization, "Approaches to the Management of HIV/AIDS in Cuba," 2004.
32. Officials from the Pan American Health Organization (PAHO) in Havana told officials at the U.S. Interests Section that "stamping ID cards used to be the case, but is no longer the practice in Cuba, something we could not independently corroborate." See "Cuban healthcare: aqui nada es facil" (nothing is easy)," confidential cable dated January 31, 2008 and released by Wikileaks, http://www.wikileaks.org/plusd/cables/08HAVANA103_a.html
33. World Health Organization, "Approaches to the Management of HIV/AIDS in Cuba," 2004.
34. Ibid.
35. Olivia Dick, Jose L. San Martin, Romeo H. Montoya, Jorgedel Diego, Betzana Zambrano, and Gustavo H. Dayan, "Review: The History of Dengue Outbreaks in the Americas," *American Journal of Tropical Medicine and Hygiene* Vol. 87, No.4 (2012), pp. 584–593.
36. Maria G. Guzman, "Thirty Years after the Cuban Dengue Hemorrhagic Epidemic of 1981," *MEDICC Review*, Vol 14, No. 2 (April 2012), translated from the Spanish and reprinted with permission from the *Revista Cubana de Medicina Tropical*, Vol. 64, No. 1 (Jan–Apr 2012).
37. Reuters, "U.S. Denies It Caused Dengue Fever in Cuba," *New York Times*, July 28, 1981.
38. "Dengue in the Americas—time to talk," *The Lancet*, Vol. 350, Issue 9076, p. 455, August 16, 1977.
39. Hirschfeld, op. cit., p. 3.
40. *The Lancet*, op. cit.
41. Hirschfeld, op. cit., p. 72.
42. Yoel Espinosa Medrano, "2013 cierran con crítica situación epidemiológica en Santa Clara," *Cubanet*, December 26, 2013.
43. Pan American Health Organization, "Epidemiological Update: Cholera," December 23, 2013.

TWO

Infrastructure and Shortages

Dr. Eloy Gonzalez, an oncologist who worked at Havana's Julio Trigo Lopez Hospital in the early 1990s, recalled a bizarre scene outside the facility during this period of worsening shortages. Food began disappearing from government-run stores and stories of people eating pet animals—their own or other people's—were circulating, though Gonzalez did not give them much credence. Then one day, while waiting for the bus outside the hospital a street vendor approached him. The man had a bag containing two dead cats, which he offered to sell the doctor.

"I was astounded," he said. Inside the hospital, shortages of supplies had forced entire wards to close, and treatment was available for only two or three cancer patients. The hospital's supplies had come from a variety of countries, with X-ray plates from the former Soviet Union, East Germany, and the Netherlands but simply stopped arriving. Workplace theft became more brazen, and Gonzalez said he observed mattresses carried out of the facility in broad daylight.[1]

The diminished economic support from the former Soviet bloc caused undeniable hardship in Cuba, yet by some accounts the worsening conditions reported during the so-called "special period in time of peace" were already being observed years earlier. Dr. Ana Solis, a pediatrician who worked at Havana's Pedro Borraz children's hospital from 1972–1980, recalls shortages of some supplies and having to search around the city for what was needed. There were some medicines and health products which had been donated from abroad, though the medical care itself "wasn't bad." The most common ailment among her young patients was asthma, aggravated by secondhand smoke. There seemed to be little awareness of the dangers of smoking among the general population at the time.[2]

According to Dr. Leonel Cordova, who worked at Havana's Joaquin Albarran Hospital, the supply of available medicines dramatically dropped during the early 1990s, and he and his colleagues often advised patients that if they couldn't fill their prescriptions at the pharmacy, they might be able to find the needed medications at the local church.

"We had to whisper this to them," he said. "We would get in trouble if we were overheard telling people to go to the church."[3] Catholic Relief Services began working on the island in 1991, sending dozens of containers of food and medicine, with much of this appropriated by government officials but at least some supplies reaching the church, which distributed them directly. Other church groups began discreetly sending medicines, health supplies and health equipment to Cuba. The Castro government's reluctant decision to develop the country's tourist industry in the 1990s also resulted in more medical donations, via tourist mules.

Not Just Tourists is a humanitarian organization started by Ken and Denise Taylor, a Canadian physician and his wife, who had been deeply moved by the medical shortages they observed during a cycling trip across Cuba in 1993. While the Cuban doctors they met seemed well-informed and competent, they had such limited access to medicines that they could offer only herbal treatments to their patients.

"One doctor told me that he hadn't had any antibiotics for his patients for two years," Taylor told *Canadian Living Magazine.*[4] Upon learning that foreign tourists were allowed to bring up to 10 kilograms of humanitarian aid into Cuba each time they visited, the couple contacted Canadian hospitals, pharmaceutical companies and other medical groups asking for donations of surplus drugs and health care products such as syringes, bandages, and surgical gloves. The Taylors set up a small warehouse where volunteers helped sort incoming contributions and filled suitcases with medicines and other medical supplies. The participating travelers were given the address of a clinic or hospital near their holiday destination, a letter in English and Spanish detailing the suitcases' contents, and explaining that they were humanitarian gifts, and a form for the recipient Cuban health care professional to sign. Many of the Canadians delivering the suitcases reported depressing conditions at the Cuban health care facilities they visited, and donations were gratefully received. One reported that

> I just delivered a suitcase in the province of Holguin in Cuba to a small clinic ("Consultorio") on the road to Gibara, a fishing village near the resort of Guardalavaca. When I opened the suitcase and they saw the content they exclaimed: "Ay, Dios mio!" ("Oh, my God!"). The nurse reached in and yanked out 2 bags with wound dressing Marian had so thoughtfully included and pressed it to her chest like a long-lost relative.
>
> Also much appreciated was the Acetaminophen (they call it Paracetamol) in all forms—Tylenol, generic—and they adored the sample

packages containing one or two pills since they can easily dispense them to patients. They had never seen those.

They say many, many thanks to each and every member of our organization. They would be happy to receive more in the future and specifically mentioned anesthetic and antibiotics. I explained that these are prescription items and may not be easily available, but even a tube of EMLA-cream would do.

They did not even have a band-aid, and no iodine either. Smaller cuts and wounds are treated with lemon juice or vinegar (ouch!!) and sutured (if necessary) without anesthetic. Only children get a shot.

Once again the hit of the season were eyeglass frames; they are literally yanked out of my hands. The grandmothers of Holguin and environs send their thank-you because now they can once again knit, read to the children, sort rice etc.[5]

Georges and Patsy Royer, a couple who earlier delivered donated medical supplies to a central collection point in eastern Cuba were able to observe some of the conditions in a local hospital when Georges got a piece of shrimp stuck in his throat:

He was very well treated and at no cost. This allowed us to see how poorly supplied this hospital was. The smaller the town, the more they need medical supplies. Patsy observed that in that particular emergency room they had no band-aids, no small gauze pads, no rubber tubing for tying off (they used a rubber glove), and the linens on the beds were in a very sad state. They were clean, but badly torn and threadbare. We also noticed that there was water running everywhere in the hospital. Not a single tap we saw would close properly, as there did not seem to be any washers in them.[6]

At a small rural clinic in eastern Cuba, the lack of a telephone line meant that in emergencies the doctor had to hail a passing vehicle in order to take patients to the hospital.[7] Another tourist was told by a hotel employee that "her mother was able to have an operation thanks to humanitarian medical donations."[8]

The Interreligious Foundation for Community Organization, also known as Pastors for Peace, arranges an annual cargo shipment of medicines, health products, and other goods to Cuba while actively campaigning for an end to U.S. trade sanctions.[9] Cuban authorities have usually welcomed such donations if delivered to government officials, but have not always been willing to cooperate with groups and individuals seeking to bring supplies directly to doctors' offices, hospitals, and clinics. Dr. Carmen Cuba Linares, a Cuban Health Ministry official who had overseen foreign medical donations, told the authors that such aid is best coordinated by government health authorities. We do not wish to be scavengers, she said.[10]

Angela Kancsal, a Canadian tourist who stayed at the Occidental Grand Playa Turquesa resort near Holguin, in eastern Cuba in 2007, brought a suitcase filled with blood pressure medication, antibiotics, and medicated creams supplied by Not Just Tourists and added her own contribution of bandages and nonprescription medications. Not Just Tourists had given her a cover letter in Spanish and English and addresses of local hospitals and clinics, but Kancsal found she had to make the delivery almost clandestinely:

> We approached a taxi and talked to him about it. He was very nervous, but took us to the village nearby. I don't think this village was used to seeing "tourists." Our first drop off was the hospital. The taxi driver asked us to wait in the car. There was a nurse standing outside, they spoke to each other and she looked around nervously and whispered to him. He told us that they cannot accept it, but told us where to go. From our understanding she wanted to take it, but could not. I believe they cannot accept "gifts" and since it was a busier location, patients, people around, maybe police? etc. It was not a choice. We went to the village doctor's office, which was literally 2 minutes away. The doctor's office was a two-room very small house. The examining table was a wooden unpadded table. The equipment was very old. My two boys could not believe it was a doctor's office. It wasn't dirty, but not completely sanitary either. When we opened up the suitcase the nurse or doctor (not sure), was overwhelmed with emotion. We were all, my family and the taxi driver overwhelmed with emotion. I am quite certain that we were the first people ever to have brought medication to them. She hugged us and was so appreciative. Kept saying we need, gracias.[11]

Denise Taylor said that in the course of her work in Not Just Tourists she had encountered two kinds of responses from Cuban officials and medical personnel—either gratitude for the help, or "deep denial" that any scarcities exist in the first place.

One doctor looked Ken [her husband] in the eye and told him, flatly, that "there are no shortages in Cuba," she recalled.[12] In 2009 the organization's Toronto office announced it was temporarily suspending shipments to Cuba. A number of travelers taking part in the program had been detained and subjected to lengthy interrogation upon arrival in Cuba, and their suitcases of donated medicines confiscated. The Toronto group said it had had unsuccessful discussions with Cuban officials, who wanted medical supplies to be sent in bulk to the island, with shipping costs paid for with funds raised by Not Just Tourists.[13]

Another group, MEMO-Cuba, has shipped redundant medical equipment and supplies no longer needed by Canadian hospitals to clinics and hospitals in Villa Clara province in central Cuba. Dr. Jerome Harvey, a physician from Thunder Bay, Ontario, first came to Cuba with a church group helping to build a children's camp and was able to visit local hospitals and speak to Cuban health professionals.

"We often say that the Cuban health care system is like a well-trained army with no weapons and no ammunition," he said. A meeting with a young doctor from Villa Clara led to the group deciding to concentrate its work in that province. The hospital in Placetas, a small city southeast of the provincial capital, was a century old, with cast iron beds from the 1930s, no functioning lab or X-ray machine and missing light switches and electrical outlets, "just bare walls," he recalled. MEMO-Cuba volunteers replaced the missing electrical fittings, but when the group returned a month later they found that these items had disappeared. Undaunted, the group brought in more electrical fittings, using epoxy glue and special screwdrivers to deter thieves.[14] MEMO-Cuba helped refurbish the hospital, whose laundry facilities consisted of a fifty-year-old Russian washing machine and whose children's outpatient clinic lacked even otoscopes and opthamascopes for examining young patients' ears and eyes.

"When we give a pediatrician an otoscope he keeps it with him, otherwise it would disappear," Harvey said. "Sometimes there isn't so much as a flashlight to look down a kid's throat."[15]

Workplace theft is not uncommon in Cuba, and by some accounts it is the main supplier of products on the black market and until recently, one of the few sources of material for the self-employed.[16] The country's health system is no exception, and according to Sergio Diaz-Briquets and Jorge Perez-Lopez, authors of *Corruption in Cuba: Castro and Beyond*, corruption in this sector "is responsible for an enormous loss of public resources and results in the denial of basic health services to needy citizens."[17] They cite the case of a radio transmitter and eight receivers which were supposed to be used by a provincial ambulance service to communicate with local hospitals but instead were installed in automobiles used by high-ranking health officials.[18] In another case, a group of at least twenty physicians were fired and barred from practicing medicine when they were discovered selling certificates prescribing special diets for diabetics, allowing the buyers to qualify for extra food rations.[19]

Low government salaries of around $20 per month are one reason for such practices, according to Diaz-Briquets. "Physicians and other health care people basically do what other Cubans do in this economy—look for ways to supplement their income," he said.[20]

There are anecdotal reports of health care personnel pilfering medicines and other supplies from hospitals to sell on the black market, and of patients bringing gifts to doctors "to get to the front of the queue or to guarantee an appointment for an X-ray, blood test or operation."[21] This practice was acknowledged even by Fidel Castro, who once told a group of foreign medical students the Cuban government was aware of "mercenaries who seek to corrupt our physicians, our health care workers, and those who will want to get under-the-table payments for providing a dental or eye consultation or some other service."[22]

Corruption in other areas of the Cuban economy also affects the provision of health care. The construction industry, with its multiple steps of planning, bidding, transport, and supply of materials, is particularly susceptible and failure to complete projects and shoddy workmanship can be blamed for some of the problems in hospitals and clinics. Julie Feinsilver author of *Healing the Masses: Cuban Health Politics at Home and Abroad,* points to the case of Havana's Frank Pais Orthopedic Hospital, where a planned expansion was underway for over a decade and a hydromassage unit only one-third complete after seven years. The hospital, whose director was on the Central Committee of the Communist Party, was considered one of Cuba's exemplary medical facilities where many foreign patients receive treatment, so one can only speculate as to the situation at other health care sites.[23] There are occasional reports in Cuba's pro-government press on this topic, and the *Havana Times,* a digital English-language newspaper (read by few Cubans), reported that the burn unit of the Calixto Garcia Hospital was still not functioning, despite having been inaugurated years earlier, and that authorities purchased "extraordinarily expensive bathtubs for burn victims, but they couldn't be used due to the low water pressure." The facility's roof had caved in on several occasions, with the Health Ministry paying repeatedly for the same botched work. The article quotes a doctor who states that in the opthamology center's warehouse "they accumulate equipment that we won't ever use and that we don't even know who ordered" and that hundreds of thousands of dollars "can be thrown away by one incompetent individual." Cement destined for projects at the Hermanos Almejeiras Hospital was used for home repairs in the Centro Havana neighborhood, "along with trucks of sand, rebar wall tile, floor tile and anything else that could be sold."[24]

Some shortages may be the result of mismanagement, with needed supplies left in warehouses and never delivered. *Granma,* the official organ of Cuba's Communist Party, reported "disorder in the distribution and control of resources" in Villa Clara province, with medical equipment and supplies lacking in some facilities stored away and gathering dust in others. Inspectors discovered thirty-seven machines for sterilizing surgical instruments, scalpels, sutures, surgical tubes, urine bags, tongue depressors, nylon gloves, stretchers, oxygen containers, Petri dishes, dental X-ray plates, fans, soap, washing machines, refrigerators, freezers, refrigerators, blankets, and 576 hospital beds. Officials were redistributing the supplies and said such abuses cost the government "million-dollar figures every year." The article warned that Cuba's state coffers were not "a bottomless barrel."[25]

In other cases Cuban customs officials confiscate materials donated directly to MINSAP, keeping them in warehouses until health ministry officials can pay import duties. Jerome Harvey recalled that a second-hand ambulance with 70,000 miles had been shipped by MEMO-Cuba but was impounded until MINSAP paid customs the equivalent of $5,000. In another incident, MEMO-Cuba, after consultations with health professionals in Villa Clara, gathered ten mammography machines and its volunteers built a mobile mammography clinic on wheels, capable of reaching Cuban women in remote areas of the province.

"Our dream was to provide breast screening for every woman in Villa Clara," he said. The mobile unit was ready but then MINSAP, without offering any explanation, told the group not to ship it. "We have written them, saying we've got this thing sitting here, we pay for shipping and so forth. Nothing, just silence. Cuban women are dying because this mobile unit is sitting in our warehouse."[26] In 2013 the charity began sending medical equipment to El Salvador, and found the process far less onerous than what it had experienced in Cuba, "like night and day."

Another disturbing feature is the high rate of hospital-acquired infections in Cuba. Patients typically bring their own bedding, food, and eating utensils, as such items are in short supply (and often pilfered), and faulty plumbing results in poor sanitation. The *Havana Times* reported that at one teaching hospital "we saw how those people accompanying the sick were wandering the corridors with receptacles full of fecal waste looking for somewhere to dispose this because the bathrooms were broken."[27] Even in the better equipped intensive care units hospital-acquired infections are common. One study published by the *International Journal of Infectious Diseases* found that 22.4 percent of ICU Cuban patients using catheters and other medical devices were affected. "DHA-HAI [device-acquired hospital infection] rates, LOS [length of stay] and mortality were found to be high, and hand hygiene low."[28]

It is difficult to reconcile the image of a modern health care system with such infrastructure problems and widespread shortages of basic supplies, which Cuban officials usually attribute to *el bloqueo,* U.S. trade sanctions. This view is expressed in a 1997 report by the American Association for World Health (AAWH), "Denial of Food and Medicine: The Impact of the U.S. Embargo on Health and Nutrition in Cuba."[29] The report praises Cuba's health system and describes some of the economic hardships in wake of the loss of Soviet trade and subsidies, especially the halving of the country's oil supply. "Medical equipment runs overtime during hours when electricity is on, and is at risk for damage with unstable voltage. Hospital air conditioning units are shut down, pharmaceutical plants produce a third of what they did in the eighties, and power outages threaten to ruin medications and vaccines in refrigerated warehouses and hospital storerooms," the report said.[30] The restricted access to U.S. medical supplies, equipment, and food had "contributed to serious nutritional deficits," "cutbacks in supplies of safe drinking water," "shortages of the most routine medical supplies," and undermined Cuban physicians' access to medical information.[31]

The AAWH report also describes the growth of U.S. pharmaceutical companies in the world market and how this expansion also hinders Cuba's access to medical supplies from other countries.[32] Dr. Jose Portilla, a health ministry official, told a group of American visitors to Havana that "we can't even import a single aspirin from Mexico."[33] Michele Frank, an American physician trained in Cuba and one of the report's contributors, told the same visitors that Cuban health officials are forced to make painful decisions as to which patients should receive life-saving treatments.[34] She called the U.S. measures "genocide," a term also used by Cuban Foreign Minister Bruno Rodriguez in addresses to the United Nations. Shortly before the U.N. General Assembly voted, for the eighteenth time, to condemn U.S. policy toward Cuba, Rodriguez said a dozen Cuban children had been forced to undergo unnecessary surgery because U.S. trade restrictions prevented their doctors from obtaining American-made catheters.[35] An oncologist in Las Tunas, a city in eastern Cuba, told a group of Finnish visitors that cancer had become the leading cause of death in the country and that "the cruel nature of the blockade" meant it was difficult to get state-of-the art equipment for radiation therapy as well as certain drugs for lung, breast, and colorectal cancers.[36]

But the U.S. trade embargo on Cuba does not cover food, telecommunications, health products and medicines or humanitarian donations, and a variety of other American products—including Colgate toothpaste, Head and Shoulders shampoo, and Jack Daniels whiskey—are sold openly in the country.[37] The 1992 Cuban Democracy Act specifically states that "exports of medicines or medical supplies, instruments, or equipment to Cuba shall not be restricted" except in cases "in which there is a reasonable likelihood that the item to be exported will be used for purposes of torture or other human rights abuses" or "in which there is a reasonable likelihood that the item to be exported will be re-exported" and cases "in which the item to be exported could be used in the production of any biotechnological product."[38] According to a partial list from the U.S. State Department's Bureau of Export Administration (BXA) between 1992 and 1998 some thirty-six licenses were issued for health care products to be exported to Cuba. These included syringes, laboratory equipment and chemicals, medical diagnostic kits, and other pharmaceutical products.[39] The Trade Sanctions Reform and Export Enhancement Act of 2000 states that the U.S. Department of Commerce "maintains a favorable licensing policy with respect to the sale and export or re-export of medicine and medical devices, food, and agricultural commodities to Cuba," while requiring payment be made by cash in advance or "by third country banks that are not U.S. persons or Government of Cuba entities."[40]

In October 1999 then-Illinois governor George Ryan visited Cuba for five days, accompanied by representatives from his state's agricultural and health care industries. After viewing the conditions in a children's hospital he told reporters the facility would be shut down if it were in his home state. Ryan met with Cuban dissidents, had a seven-hour meeting with Fidel Castro, and negotiated permission for a seven-year old Cuban boy with liver disease to leave the country for medical treatment in North Carolina, where he had relatives.[41]

A few months after Ryan's visit, Havana's PABEXPO international conference center was the site of a four-day U.S. health care exhibition, the first American trade show in Cuba since the 1959 revolution. An estimated 8,000 Cuban medical professionals toured the product displays of 97 U.S. health companies, including Proctor and Gamble, Eastman Kodak, Archer Daniels Midland, and a California-based subsidiary of a German optical and electronics company already selling $1 million in products annually to Cuba through its headquarters in Germany. The companies handed out samples of medicines and vitamins, and donated most of the products they had brought (including a radiation therapy machine worth $365,000) as a goodwill gesture. Cuban officials from MediCuba, the state agency responsible for medical imports, described the exhibit as a "tremendous success," while several American company representatives reported serious inquiries about their products.[42]

The following year there was a second visit to Cuba by Governor Ryan and representatives of some of the health exhibitors, which the Americans were hoping would result in contracts. Jeff Dziura, then international sales director for the wound care products firm Ferris Manufacturing Company, said there were meetings with Cuban health officials at Havana's Hotel Nacional that were more focused than previous contacts had been and they were given a tour of several Havana hospitals. At a clinic for edema and ulcer sufferers he was surprised to find patients treated with "mud baths in the sun." At another hospital the lab was little more than a hallway, and test tubes were topped with cotton rather than stoppers.

The delegation was invited to dinner with both Fidel and Raul Castro and found the experience intimidating. Dziura recalled that Raul was very quiet during the eight-course dinner but that Fidel Castro delivered "a long rant" and proved himself very knowledgeable about Illinois corn. He showed his guests the buffalo milk he drank and sharply ordered a wine steward with a trolley to leave, as if he did not want his guests to see the selection of wines. Castro dismissed the representative of a larger health care company, telling him he "had too many products" but questioned Dziura at length about his firm. The American executive said he couldn't really ask any questions of Castro, but that after the dinner two other Cuban officials approached him to say there was genuine interest in Medecines San Frontiére's wound care products. Dziura said his contact with the Cubans continued for a time, then stopped abruptly in wake of former president George Bush's hardline Cuba speech on May 20, 2002. "The Iron Curtain came down," he recalled.[43]

At least one of the Illinois-based health care companies did make some sales to Cuba following Governor Ryan's visit. Baxter International manufactures products to treat a variety of acute and chronic diseases such as hemophilia and immune disorders. According to a company spokeswoman, "on occasion Baxter has exported and/or donated critical, lifesaving medical products to Cuba over the years in accordance with government policies and regulations, but not in any sustained or meaningful manner/amount."[44]

American agricultural exports to Cuba did not suffer during this period. For a few months after Bush's speech Havana's PABEXPO center hosted the U.S. Food and Agribusiness Exhibition for the second year in a row and authorized food exports from the United States have grown steadily, reaching $457.3 million in 2012. The value of U.S. medical supplies, instruments, equipment, and pharmaceutical products authorized for export to Cuba in recent years has fluctuated from $85,000 in 2009 to $2.2 million in 2013, according to the New York-based U.S.-Cuba Trade and Economic Council, which provided the following figures, as shown in Table 2.1.

But there are political and economic factors influencing Cuba's decisions on whether or not to buy American products. According to the Council, in 2007 officials from Alimport, the Cuban government agency in charge of food imports, told representatives of U.S.-based companies that it would significantly reduce purchases from their firms "due to a lack of effort (and, presumably success) by United States-based companies in obtaining changes to United States laws and United States regulations."[45] In other words, would-be U.S. exporters were expected to lobby Washington on Cuba's behalf.

Many medical products are purchased more cheaply in other countries, and Cuba has imported stethoscopes and MRI machines from China, its second largest trading partner, which offered Cuba a $70 million credit for health infrastructure during Hu Jintao's visit to the island in 2008. Other sources of medicines and medical supplies include Brazil,

Table 2.1.

Year	Value of U.S. medical supplies, instruments, equipment, and pharmaceutical products authorized for export to Cuba
2009	US$85,408.00
2010	US$226,563.00
2011	US$103,771.00
2012	US$200,630.00
2013	US$2.2 million

Argentina, Mexico and Germany. The president of Cuba's oncology society, Lorenzo Anasagasti, has been quoted as saying that Cuba sends undercover buyers to the United States "to buy everything we need" and carry the supplies back without permits. The buyers "are blond, with blue eyes" and "they even speak good English."[46]

Some Cuban health facilities, especially those catering to foreigners, are clean and well-equipped and often impress visitors. A Canadian traveler who stayed with his family at the Sirinis La Salina resort in Varadero, which had its own medical clinic with a doctor and nurse, described it as "pristine." When his wife became ill, the doctor diagnosed overexposure to the sun compounded by an allergic reaction to sunscreen, gave her a cortisone injection and calamine lotion, and wrote out a prescription which the nurse delivered to their room in less than thirty minutes. The couple was charged 140 convertible pesos or CUCs (or US $140) and given a receipt for their insurance provider.[47]

The Centro de Investigaciones Médico Quirúgicas (CIMEQ) in Havana is one of Cuba's best hospitals, and believed to be the facility where the late Venezuelan president Hugo Chavez received part of his treatment for cancer during several visits. The hospital's website posts photographs showing modern equipment and well-appointed rooms and lists fifteen different medical services, including liver, pancreas, kidney, cornea and bone marrow transplants, obesity, and cancer treatments plus fourteen different cosmetic surgical procedures.

"Notable personalities from the arts, sciences and politics from all parts of the world have received attention in its modern and functional installations," the site says. "It has a Latin American Center for Medical Events where each year innumerable scientific activities are held."[48] For patients arriving from outside Cuba, CIMEQ offers ambulance service from the airport.

There is some question as to whether Chavez was treated at CIMEQ, as there was little outward indication of increased security at the hospital, and patients consulted reported seeing no Cuban secret service agents on the premises.[49] While CIMEQ is known to treat members of Cuba's political elite, there is another private facility, the Kohly clinic, reportedly used by the Castros themselves and located not far from Fidel's residence in western Havana.

The Clinica Central Cira Garcia, also located in western Havana, markets its services to foreigners via Cubanacan, the Cuban state tourism agency, and offers treatment packages such as a comprehensive medical check-up with a one-night stay for 575 CUCs, an outpatient battery of tests and examinations for infants up to two years old for 495 CUCs, and a twenty-one-night program for multiple sclerosis patients for 5,016 CUCs.[50] And a Cuban travel agency offered cancer patients a regime of homeopathic treatments in seven, fifteen, and twenty-one-day stays with accommodation at the Hotel Club Acuario located on Havana's Hemingway Marina. Billed as "the first Touristic Package designed to provide homeopathic natural oncological treatment," the program includes a city tour of Old Havana with a professional guide, medical consultations, and a combination of four Cuban nutritional and homeopathic remedies.[51]

Cuban officials clearly view health tourism as a new and important source of revenue in an economy still recovering from the loss of subsidies from the former Soviet Union and battered by hurricane damage. Since 2010 Cuba has required foreign visitors to have health insurance, and pay for any medical treatment in hard currency, with some health insurance policies sold by the Cuban state. While more paying foreigners arrive at Cuban hospitals and clinics, the medical system used by Cubans continues to suffer as public payrolls are cut and a 12 percent reduction in the health budget is imposed. In 2010 the country closed 54 hospitals and hundreds of smaller family clinics, reducing the number of medical facilities from 13,203 to 12,738, a decline of 3.5 percent. The patient load for family doctors has increased from an average of 120–160 families to 300–400 families. The government also began a campaign called "health care is free but how much does it cost?" in an effort to increase public awareness of state health care expenditures. The campaign represented something of a political shift in the way health care is presented, from a universal right to a service that must be financed.

NOTES

1. Interview with Dr. Eloy Gonzalez, December 11, 2013.
2. Interview with Dr. Ana Solis, June 25, 2013.
3. Interview with Dr. Leonel Cordova, August 15, 2013.
4. Hasulo, Susanne, *Canadian Living Salutes: Denise and Ken Taylor*, http://canadianliving.com/life/community. Accessed September 15, 2009.
5. From an account by Brigit Nagy, posted December 2007, in "Suitcase Stories," posted on the Not Just Tourists/Plus que touristes website, http://www.njt-pqt.org. Accessed on March 5, 2011.
6. From an account by Georges and Patsy Royer, op. cit.
7. From an account by Karen Weatherbe, posted on http://www.njttoronto.ca/experiences3.htm. Accessed January 10, 2010. "The clinic is a small rural one—no telephone line—in case of an emergency the Dr. needs to flag down a truck or car to take his patients to the hospital in Chivirico. We have been friends of Dr. Ricardo Suarez (doctor) and his wife Dr. Odolys Vargas (dentist) for about 5 years. I was touched when the Dr. already knew who would benefit from the supplies we took. A patient was really in need of a back brace we had taken."
8. Ibid.
9. The organization's website invites readers to "see Cuba for Yourself and Challenge the U.S. Blockade!" http://www.ifconews.org/node/948.
10. Interview in Miami with Dr. Carmen Cuba Linares, September 1, 2010.
11. Email correspondence with Angela Kancsal. The author traveled to Cuba in November of 2012 with Global Exchange, which suggested tour members bring donations of over-the-counter medicines and other health supplies, but to spread them around in our luggage—a tacit indication that such donations are sometimes confiscated at the airport.

12. Interview with Denise Taylor, June 12, 2013.
13. From www.notjusttourists.org. Accessed April 21, 2010. An earlier notice posted on the website, dated December 1, 2009, said that the organization was "quite hopeful that the problems we have experienced in the past year at Cuban Customs are close to being resolved."
14. Written correspondence with Dr. Jerome Harvey, June 24, 2013.
15. Interview with Dr. Jerome Harvey, June 24, 2013.
16. The private wholesale market did not open in Cuba until March of 2013, with a pilot project on Isla de la Juventud to see food products, consumer and industrial goods. See "Cuba opens wholesale market for private business," *Agence France-Presse* report, March 7, 2013.
17. Sergio Diaz-Briquets and Jorge Perez-Lopez, *Corruption in Cuba: Castro and Beyond* (Austin: University of Texas Press, 2006), p. 44.
18. Ibid., p. 133.
19. Ibid., p. 136.
20. Interview with Sergio Diaz-Briquets, July 5, 2013.
21. Lucia Newman, "The Truths and Tales of Cuban Healthcare," http://www.aljazeera.com/indepth/features/2012/06/201265115527622647.html.
22. From a speech given by Fidel Castro at the Escuela Latinoamericana de Medicina, December 3, 2002. Quoted in Diaz-Briquets and Perez-Lopez, op. cit., p 136.
23. Julie Feinsilver, *Healing the Masses: Cuban Health Politics at Home and Abroad* (Berkeley: University of California Press, 1993), p 204.
24. Fernando Ravsberg, "Cuba's Health Resources Dilemma," *Havana Times*, April 29, 2010. http://www.havanatimes.org/?p=23499.
25. *Granma*, February 26, 2010, accessed March 2, 2010.
26. Jerome Harvey, op. cit.
27. Ravsberg, op. cit.
28. H. Guanche-Garcell, V. D. Requejo-Pino O Rosenthal, C. Morales-Perez, O. Delgado-Gonzalez, and D. Fernandez-Gonzalez, "Device-associated infection rates in adult intensive care units of Cuban university hospitals: International Nosocomial Infection Control Consortium (INICC) findings." *International Journal of Infectious Diseases*, May 2011.
29. American Association for World Health, "Denial of Food and Medicine: The Impact of the U.S. Embargo on Health and Nutrition in Cuba," March 1997. http://www.medicc.org/resources/documents/embargo/The%20impact%20of%20the%20U.S.%20Embargo%20on%20Health%20&%20Nutrition%20in%20Cuba.pdf.
30. Ibid., p 37.
31. Ibid., "Summary of Findings."
32. Ibid., pp. 12–14.
33. Statement made by Dr. Jose Portilla to a group of American visitors (including the author) at the International Friendship Institute in Havana, November 12, 2012.
34. From a presentation given by Michele Frank in Havana on November 17, 2012 at which the author was present.
35. Will Weisert, "Embargo as Genocide? US disputes Cuban claim," *Associated Press*, December 4, 2009.
36. Remarks by Dr. Juan Ernesto Perez Reyes as reported in *Periodico 26*, June 28, 2013, http://www.periodico26.cu/index.php/en/principal-es-2/9635-finnish-solidarity-brigade-learns-about-impacts-of-us-blockade-on-healthcare.
37. Author's observations during a trip to Cuba in November 2012. In addition to the products mentioned, apples from Virginia and Coca-Cola (bottled in Mexico) were also on sale.
38. Office of Foreign Assets Control (OFAC), "Cuba: What You Need to Know About U.S. Sanctions Against Cuba," updated January 24, 2012.http://www.treasury.gov/resource-center/sanctions/Programs/Documents/cuba.pdf.
39. From the Section 6004 of the Cuban Democracy Act, http://www.treasury.gov/resource-center/sanctions/Documents/cda.pdf.

40. Economic Eye on Cuba, 4 May 1998–10 May 1998, http://www.cubatrade.org/eyeonv.html.

41. "George Ryan in Cuba: Seven Hours with Fidel," *The Economist*, October 28, 1999.

42. Economic Eye on Cuba, 24 January–30 January, 2000, http://www.cubatrade.org/eyeonv.html.

43. Interview with Jeff Dziura, June 28, 2012.

44. Written correspondence from Baxter International External Communications Department, September 9, 2013.

45. "2012–2001 U.S. Export Statistics for Cuba," Economic Eye on Cuba, February 2013, U.S.-Cuba Trade and Economic Council, New York.

46. Weisert, op. cit.

47. Written correspondence dated January 3, 2012, from a Canadian traveler who asked that his family's privacy be respected.

48. http://www.cimeq.org/es/.

49. Rodriguez, Andrea, "Chavez reportedly at exclusive Cuba hospital," Associated Press, January 17, 2013.

50. http://www.cirag.cu/ingles/index.htm.

51. http://cuba-yes.com/en/health/cancer-medical-package.php.

THREE

Women and Children

The Necropolis de Colon in Havana is one of the largest cemeteries in the Americas, and among its most visited sites is the tomb of *La Milagrosa*, the miraculous one. It holds the remains of Amelia Goiry de la Hoz, a wealthy young woman who died in childbirth in 1903. Her baby died shortly afterwards and was placed at her feet in the same coffin. Her inconsolable husband visited daily, bringing flowers and making a ritual of tapping the gravestone, asking her to wake up. The legend holds that when her grave was opened, Amelia's corpse was holding her baby. The large sculpture atop the tomb is made of Tuscan marble and shows a woman holding a baby with her left arm, and in her right hand, a cross—a symbol of sacrifice.

Cubans make the pilgrimage to the tomb to ask this unofficial saint to protect their health and that of family and friends. Conditions for women and children have greatly improved since *La Milagrosa's* time, and the charity Save the Children, using official Cuban health statistics, has ranked Cuba as the best country in Latin America and among developing nations in which to be a mother.[1] Nevertheless, motherhood can still be a precarious undertaking in Cuba and women are having fewer babies than ever. The country has undergone a dramatic drop in birth rates, from an average of 4.18 births per woman in 1960, the year after the Revolution, to 1.46 in 2012.[2]

Some scholars have pointed out that Cuba's birth rate began to decline before the Revolution, with fertility levels in the 1950s approaching those of developed countries. There was an increase in births in the early 1960s, reaching a high of 35.1 per thousand population in 1963, perhaps caused by some hopes of a more prosperous future during the early years of the Revolution.[3] But the following year the birth rate began to fall, edging downward, to less than ten per thousand in 2011 and seems likely to remain below replacement levels for the immediate future.

The health of babies and children under five has been an oft-stated priority of the Castro government, which frequently points to a lower infant mortality rate than that of the United States.[4] This official figure has been challenged by some analysts, who have noted statistical anomalies such as a relatively high maternal death rate, a phenomenon which will be discussed later in this chapter. But first we will examine Cuba's health programs for women and children and the social and environmental settings in which they are practiced.

The legal age of sexual consent in Cuba is sixteen, and according to Yasmany Diaz of the country's Centro Nacional de Educación Sexual (CENESEX), a recent census indicated that the average age at which Cubans begin sexual activity (though not necessarily intercourse) has gone down in recent years to ages thirteen to fourteen. Condoms and intrauterine devices are the most frequent forms of birth control rather than injectable hormonal contraceptives and the pill, which he said were not used much due to U.S. *bloqueo,* nor the morning after pill (though these products are also manufactured by European and Asian pharmaceutical companies). There is no explicit sex education until ages ten to eleven, when the subject—including condom use and HIV/AIDS prevention—is incorporated into civic education classes.[5]

The reported behavior of young Cubans suggests that the information contained in these classes is not always put to use, even in the case of academic high achievers. A study published in the country's public health journal, the *Revista Cubana de Salud Publica* surveyed fifteen- to nineteen-year-olds enrolled in preuniversity programs in Havana and Holguin on their knowledge of HIV/AIDS and condom use and found that

> Of the total number of students, 54.6 percent did not use any condom in their first sexual intercourse whereas roughly 50 percent admitted that they used it occasionally with both fixed and occasional partners. Also, 34.5 percent of students had kept their regular partners during the last year and 23.9 percent had had two or three partners; the rest only had a very small number—four or more partners. It called the attention that some young people stated that they had had 20 partners and others were incapable of mentioning an exact figure. It was considered that 2.7 percent had high risk of acquiring AIDS.[6]

Cuba produces some of its own condoms, imports others from Korea and China, and receives some donated condoms from international organizations. But periodic shortages of condoms (along with supplies of many goods) are occasionally reported in the Cuban press. On January 1, 2013, a columnist for *Juventud Rebelde,* the newspaper of Cuba's Union of Young Communists, wrote that a reader had informed him that for over a year there had been no fifteen-centavo condoms in any of the pharmacies in the city of Santa Clara, a provincial capital in central Cuba, and that since November there had been none of the higher quality one-peso condoms, except a few past their expiration dates. A second reader reported a similar situation in the eastern city of Holguin.[7]

The following year another Cuban newspaper, *Vanguardia*, in the central province of Villa Clara, reported an increase in syphilis cases in the region, along with an increase in women seeking abortions, "a decision which conspires against the need to increase the birth rate in the most aging province of the country."[8] The article said that condoms had virtually disappeared from local pharmacies and that one million condoms imported from China were being retained in a warehouse until they could be relabelled with the "correct" expiration date of December 2014. The newspaper did not publish the original (and presumably, much earlier) expiration date, but cited a letter from the Cuban Health Ministry, dated July 9, 2012, authorizing the change. As there was a shortage of personnel to relabel the condoms, pharmacies were allowed to sell the Chinese prophylactics in the original packaging, but were required to explain the situation.[9]

Injectable hormonal contraceptives have been used on a limited basis, and Cuban researchers have published at least two studies on their efficacy and side effects. An article in *Revista Cubana de Obstetricia y Ginecologia* describes a study of 103 women who voluntarily tried Noristerat, produced by the Germany pharmaceutical company Bayer, from 1989 to 1994. The study's authors reported that none of the patients became pregnant, that most liked the method and wanted to continue using the injectable contraceptive and that only two suffered side effects.[10]

Another study examined the effects of the injectable contraceptive Depo-Provera on glucose metabolism in twenty-one women aged twnty to thirty-five. The team of researchers from Cuba's Instituto Nacional de Endocrinologia reported alterations after three and nine months of use, "which, although statistically significant, does not reach clinical importance."[11] Interestingly, Depo-Provera is produced by a U.S. pharmaceutical company, Pfizer, though presumably the study's authors had no trouble accessing the drug.

The official figure for contraceptive prevalence—the percentage of women who are practicing, or whose sexual partners are practicing, any form of contraception—is 74 percent, the highest in Latin America and the Caribbean and Cuban authorities have predicted this figure would reach 80 percent by 2015.[12] But there are indications that abortion is still frequently used as a birth control method, as was the case in prerevolutionary Cuba.

Most forms of abortion were prohibited in Cuba until 1938, when the procedure was made legal in cases of rape and where pregnancy threatened the woman's life or where "hereditary or contagious conditions threatened to cause fetal birth defects or disease." Only the most privileged women would have had access to contraceptives, and illegal abortions were still widely practiced—by some accounts available "on demand and at a very low cost for those who could not afford a steep fee."[13] Ironically, access to abortion may have been reduced in the first few years following the revolution, as the vice network which controlled gambling, prostitution, and illegal abortions was broken up. Cuba's pool of physicians shrank and those who remained became more reluctant to perform the procedure. There was an increase in mortality from self-induced abortions, prompting the Ministry of Public Health to loosen restrictions in 1965, permitting elective abortions in pregnancies of up to ten weeks' gestation and afterwards for medical reasons. Five years later a study revealed that many Cuban women were still suffering from the after effects of self-induced abortions and authorities began to publicize the dangers of the practice and increase efforts to promote the use of contraceptives.[14] The government later drafted a new Penal Code making abortion a crime if practiced for profit, performed outside a medical institution, or by nonspecialized personnel or without the consent of the pregnant woman—provisions aimed at further discouraging illegal abortions.

The influence of the Catholic Church on abortion and contraceptive practice in Cuba appears to be very limited, and a study by Canadian researchers noted a striking absence of religious considerations among women seeking abortions in Cuba. In 2005, Danièle Bélanger and Andrea Flynn interviewed twenty-four women who had undergone at least one abortion and ten men whose partners had an abortion. "Even for respondents reporting that their families were highly religious, the personal decision to terminate a pregnancy was not seen as contentious on religious or moral grounds," they reported. One Cuban physician mentioned a "*cultura abortiva*" to the researchers, while another stated that abortion was used habitually and viewed as unproblematic.

"In reference to some of her patients, one doctor said, "they have friends who have obtained ten abortions without any problems," Bélanger and Flynn wrote. "This statement supports our interview evidence of the importance of personal networks in influencing individuals' views on abortion."[15]

In wake of Pope John Paul II's visit in 1998, Fidel Castro said that abortion should not be used as a form of birth control, which might pose health risks. He called for better sex education and said that Cuba did not "have to go back to the Middle Ages and invent the chastity belt again."[16] That same year a dissident Cuban doctor wrote a survey of abortion practices at the Hospital Materno-Infantil 10 de Octubre in Havana, charging that patients undergoing second trimester abortions had not had the procedure explained to them, were not advised of potential complications, and that in at least seven cases, living fetuses with no malformations were left to die. Dr. Oscar Elias Biscet sent his report directly to

Fidel Castro, and was almost immediately arrested and sent to prison for three years.[17]

While abortion numbers have declined, Cuba still has one of the highest abortion rates in the world, 24.8 per thousand women aged fifteen to forty-four, behind Russia (53.7), Kazakhstan (35), Estonia (33.3), Belarus (31.7) and Latvia 27.3), according to United Nations population figures.[18] The practice remains the preferred form of birth control for many Cuban women. A Cuban survey of over 4,200 pregnant women published in 2006 included 1,806 who were terminating their pregnancies. Of this subset, 52.2 percent reported they had been using, then abandoned, some form of contraception; another 30.1 percent professed a lack of knowledge of contraceptive methods, and 7.3 percent indicated they preferred abortion over contraception. Repeat abortions were common, with 16.3 percent reporting two or more previous abortions.[19] The Canadian researchers Bélanger and Flynn also found widespread "skepticism and negative perceptions" about contraceptive methods which undermined their effective use and "sometimes precluded the practice of contraception altogether." In addition, there were concerns about side effects. Several of their respondents had suffered pain and infections while using IUDs, and expressed doubts over the effectiveness of condoms, which were viewed mostly as a way to avoid sexually transmitted disease.[20]

The quality and availability of contraceptives seems likely to be a factor as well. Dr. Alberto Dominguez-Bali, a Miami-based obstetrician and gynecologist whose practice includes recently arrived Cuban immigrants, said many of these patients had multiple cervical lacerations and that 30 to 40 percent had undergone more than two abortions. A number of Cuban women had had IUDs implanted without their knowledge, and some had two IUDs—one inserted without their knowledge and another inserted upon their request. He said some of the intrauterine devices removed were of a type no longer used in most countries, including the notorious Dalkon Shield (found to cause injury to a disproportionately large number of its users, withdrawn from the market in the United States in 1974 and the subject of over 300,000 lawsuits). Other patients had rustic handmade IUDs formed out of metal and fishing line, and in one case, a small chicken bone and fishing line. Many of the devices had very short strings, making their removal impossible without a hysteroscopy.

Dominguez-Bali also observed widespread misconceptions among these patients, such as the belief that the pill and injectable contraceptives caused facial hair or breast cancer. Most were unwilling to use hormonal types of birth control, he said, adding that the diaphragm was also unknown to his Cuban patients.[21]

Cuba's abortion figures do not include the number of women undergoing menstrual extraction, a procedure performed within forty-five days of a patient's last period. The practice was first offered in 1968, as part of a revamped national health care program for women. Women over eighteen do not need to have a pregnancy confirmed in order to undergo the procedure, but approximately two-thirds are believed to result in the termination of pregnancy.[22] There are no published statistics on *regulacion menstrual*, but health authorities are sufficiently concerned to issue warnings to young Cuban women on its potential complications. Dr. Rafael Abreu Naranjo, a gynecologist and obstetrician, told the Cuban youth magazine *Somos Jovenes* that while menstrual extraction was less risky than abortion, both procedures could result in "uterine perforation, internal genital infections, blood loss, anemia, among others which put at risk future fertility and occasionally even life."[23]

Cuban women wanting to bear babies are quickly incorporated into the Programa Nacional de Atención Materno-Infantil Prenatal (PAMI), the maternal-infant program that is perhaps the best-funded health care provision in the country. Pregnant women undergo an average of twelve prenatal visits and receive extra food rations, including milk and are supposed to receive nutritional supplements—though the actual availability of these items varies.[24] The patient's family physician is required to carry out a thorough intake exam no later than the ninth week of pregnancy and blood samples are taken to test alpha-feto protein levels, which could indicate neural tube defects or other anomalies. Ultrasound has been available in many polyclinics since 2003, when Fidel Castro announced that the service was being inaugurated in thirty-one facilities in Havana and another twenty-six in other provinces.[25] If a pregnant woman misses an appointment, her physician is likely to visit her in her home.

While Cuban authorities have made maternal-infant care a priority, the programs are also affected by the health care system's deteriorating infrastructure. An account by a U.S. Foreign Service medical officer in a confidential cable released by Wikileaks offers a glimpse of conditions in some Cuban ob/gyn facilities. The unnamed official accompanied a pregnant staff member of the U.S. Interests Section to an appointment with a highly recommended physician at the Hospital Ginecobstétrico Ramón González Coro, a 300-bed specialist hospital for pregnant women in the Vedado section of Havana.

> At the nursing station there was no nurse, but a metal cabinet with glass doors that had one jar filled with cotton and one half-full 16 ounce bottle of isopropyl alcohol. There were no other supplies nor any indication this was a nurse's station—no stethoscopes, no computers, no medical charts, no papers or pens on the desk—there was a lone dial-type black telephone. After waiting 15 minutes a nurse in a white uniform appeared and told the FSHP and her patient to wait. She wasn't friendly. There was no waiting room, so they found some chairs in the hall. It was very hot and the patient was very anxious and in pain. After 45 minutes and several attempts in a polite manner to move

> things along, a young female doctor came out smiling and asked for the patient—she asked that her husband remain in the chair, but did allow the FSHP to go with her upon insisting.
>
> The American visitors were guided to the second floor, reserved for foreigners and supposedly the nicest part of the hospital, and to an examining room which was empty except for "only one old rusting sheet-metal table without any covering, extensions or stirrups." The American health professional brought paper drapes to cover the table and the patient, while the Cuban physician used an old Pinard fetal heart stethoscope, a device similar to an ear trumpet that was developed in the nineteenth century, to listen to the baby's heart beat. The cable reported that the doctor, while clinically competent, seemed abrupt and rough with the patient. "She stated, 'She has an infection and needs an antibiotic,' and gave the FSHP a written prescription for an antibiotic generally not recommended during pregnancy." Upon returning to the U.S. Interests Section's health unit, the American medical professional did a lab culture whose results indicated the pregnant patient did not in fact have an infection. "As a result of this experience, the FSHP concluded that the best care for her unstable female pregnant patients in Havana—barring a MEDEVAC to the U.S.—would be by the FSHP in their own home with telephone consults to an obstetrician in the U.S."[26]

Pregnant women who are deemed at risk are sometimes sent to maternity homes, residences where their health is monitored and food intake ensured and where they can more easily access specialized obstetric care. Maternity homes have been used in Europe, North America, and many developing countries to accommodate women living in remote areas during their final weeks of pregnancy, ensuring their access to a hospital when it is time to give birth, and are credited with reducing both maternal and infant mortality. The first maternity homes were opened in 1962 in eastern Cuba, a year after the national health service was established, and by 1989 accounted for nearly 30 percent of all births.[27] The maternity homes were set up in buildings constructed for other purposes, and while their programs and organization vary, all have kitchens and common rooms where residents may participate in recreational activities and attend classes on childcare. Larger maternity homes have a full-time physician on staff, and a nurse is supposed to be in attendance around the clock. The women's blood pressure and other vital signs are recorded on a daily basis, and this information incorporated into their medical records. There is no data on how many pregnant women refuse referrals to maternity homes, but one study cited by the World Health Organization (WHO) found that in 1989 about 9 percent of women left the residences before giving birth.[28] In general, the maternity homes were viewed as a successful program and over the years expanded to 338 such facilities, though subsequent government cutbacks reduced the number of maternity homes to 143 in 2011.[29]

In the past most pregnant women living in remote areas were referred to maternity homes after the thirty-fourth week of gestation, but today nutritional deficiencies are among the most frequent reasons for the referrals. One study of 150 pregnant women in Havana found that their average calorie, carbohydrate, and protein consumption was below the recommended level, and there were shortfalls in thiamine, folic acid, and niacin, among other deficiencies.[30] Another report compiled by the United Nations Development Program and the Cuban Health Ministry reported anemia in 24 percent of third-trimester pregnant women and 12 percent of this group was also underweight.[31] If these figures are correct (and not an underestimate of nutritional deficits, as critics might suspect) it still seems obvious that the supply of vitamin and mineral supplements is insufficient and there may not be enough maternity homes in the country to accommodate every patient in need of this service.

Elise Andaya, who studied Cuba's reproductive health services during thirteen months of research in Havana for her dissertation from 2004–2005, reported that Cuban television often broadcast programs on maternity homes in which the women residents praised the care they received and the high quality of the food. But family doctors often told pregnant women "in the form of a good-natured, but serious threat" that they could be sent to a maternity home if their health indicators failed to improve. One doctor agreed with her patient that conditions in some maternity homes were depressing, and many women did not like being separated from their families. Andaya describes the following doctor-patient exchange:

> On another occasion, I sat with Janet as she examined a slender young woman in her second trimester whose weight gain fell below the desired norms. Frowning, she asked, "Are you eating well?" When the woman responded in the affirmative, Janet shook her head again, slightly disbelievingly, and declared her intention to refer her to a maternity home. Met with the woman's violent protestations, Janet relented, but declared, "I'll give you two weeks to gain the weight, otherwise you're going straight to the maternity home." After the patient departed, Janet told me she believed that the woman was sharing many of the additional rations of her prenatal diet—particularly the dairy allotments—with her child who, having just turned seven years old, had recently become ineligible for the additional dairy rations provided to young children.[32]

Nutritional deficiencies are partly the result of Cuban agriculture's chronically poor production—the country imports over 70 percent of its food—as well as cultural attitudes regarding food. Cuba has the fourth highest per capita sugar consumption in the world, and prior to the so-called Special Period, obesity had been a serious health concern, affecting more women than men. By the mid-1990s obesity levels began to rebound and by 2010 exceeded pre-crisis levels.[33] There have been periodic campaigns to improve nutrition, and a 1983 pamphlet published the Ministry of Public Health urged Cubans to exercise more.[34] But the traditional Cuban diet is dominated by rice, beans, pork, and relatively few fruits and vegetables, along with high levels of sugar consumption, and a 2001 survey revealed food preferences seemingly unaffected by any government dietary warnings and influenced by a limited selection of available items.

There was almost no consumption of whole grain cereals, and 90 percent of respondents indicated they would eat fried foods at every meal if they could, including butter, bacon, and pork cracklings. Half of those surveyed consumed over 20 percent of their daily calories in sugar, and over 90 percent said they would like to have soft drinks at every meal. Research at the Institute of Nutrition and Food Hygiene undertaken the following year revealed that half of Cubans surveyed did not relate diet to health, that 25 percent were unaware of cholesterol's damaging effect on health. Almost all respondents (98 percent) believed meat should be eaten every day, with red meat considered to be the healthiest. Ham was believed to be a very good food for children, and 85 percent would feed their children ham every day if possible.[35]

Some Cuban nutritionists recommend sugar as part of a daily diet for underweight pregnant women. One *consulta de nutrición* posted by a dissident Cuban blogger listed four tablespoons of sugar, four tablespoons of marmalade, and a tablespoon of mayonnaise as part of a pregnant woman's prescribed daily diet, along with beans, rice, meat, yogurt, fruit, and vegetables plus a cup of coffee in the morning.[36]

Another unhealthy element is the country's high level of tobacco consumption. According to the 2001 Second National Survey on Risk Factors and Chronic Diseases, 22.3 percent of Cuban women smoke (compared with 39.9 percent of Cuban men), with the habit more prevalent among those over forty, of African descent and "with a perceived economic situation as very poor." Another national study published almost a decade later reported little decline in smoking levels, and observed that over half the Cuban population was exposed to secondhand smoke: 55 percent of children, 51 percent of pregnant women, and 60 percent of adolescents.[37]

Until the 1990s all Cubans over eighteen received a monthly ration of cigarettes, but this provision continued for those fifty-five and older until 2010. The measure allowed Cubans to buy eighty cigarettes per month for the equivalent of about 30 cents, using their ration books at state-run stores, though most smokers consumed far more than this amount, often buying cigarettes from nonsmokers at twice the price. The move to end the tobacco ration seems to have been motivated more by economic necessity than concerns about public health, and official Cuban government policy on smoking seems ambivalent. Anti-smoking messages in the country do not carry the dire warnings seen in other countries; one public announcement spotted by the author said that "smoking harms sexual potency and fertility." Cuba's state tobacco company produces a cigar aimed at women smokers, the Julieta, although much of the country's famous cigar industry is aimed at foreign buyers. Most Cuban smokers consume domestic-made cigarettes, which are usually filterless and contain a harsh dark tobacco, which has been linked to the country's high rate of mouth, larynx, and esophagus cancers, as well as lung cancer. The habit is prevalent even among health professionals, and doctors and nurses taking cigarette breaks are a common sight outside Cuban hospitals. A 2007 survey of over 700 medical staff in Habana Vieja revealed that 36.4 percent smoked, and that among women in the health care field who smoked, 36.7 continued to do so even during pregnancy.[38]

Almost all births take place in hospitals, and Cuba is one of the few countries in the world that still does not allow fathers in the delivery room, although they may be with the mother in the hospital during the first stage of labor.[39] A study of thirty-six women giving birth in three Havana hospitals by researchers from the University of Havana's biology department and the Escuela Nacional de Salud Pública stated, bluntly, that "knowledge about pregnancy, childbirth and postpartum in Cuba is currently deficient," and that giving birth in the country's hospitals can be a demeaning experience, in which few of the recommendations by WHO for appropriate interventions during childbirth are followed.[40]

The first WHO recommendation states that "the well-being of the new mother must be ensured through free access of a chosen member of her family during birth and throughout the postnatal period. In addition, the health team must provide emotional support."[41] Most of the women in the study wanted their own mothers to be present and told the researchers that their babies' fathers were not prepared for the event. They did express a desire for the fathers to be with them in the recovery room, but this was not allowed. During labor the women "were left with their gowns open, exposed to both medical and nonmedical personnel" with no sheets to cover themselves. The researchers observed that hospital staff rarely used the term "señora" when addressing the women, and tended to use diminutive expressions which might be more appropriate with a child, such as "*mamita, mija, mijita, mi chiquitica, negrita.*"[42]

Each woman was given an IV, most were connected to a fetal monitor and subjected to an artificial rupture of membranes, which WHO guidelines discourage as routine procedures. All the women were made to adopt the lithotomy position, lying on their backs, feet raised above the hips, the most common but least comfortable position as it puts pressure on the vaginal walls, works against gravity, and can reduce oxygen flow to the fetus. Other practices going against WHO recommendations included routine episiotomies (undertaken in twenty-nine of the thirty-six cases studied), and one of the obstetricians told the researchers that it was much easier to suture an incision than a vaginal tear. But most of the women found the experience traumatic, and were not given any explanation for the procedures to which they were subjected (WHO guidelines say that "women must participate in decisions about their birth experiences"[43]). When asked about this situation one of the obstetricians expressed annoyance. "Just imagine having to repeat to each one of them what is being done and why it is being done." In the researchers' view, "the routine use of some medical interventions and the institutional regulations described are manifestations of physical and gender violence."[44]

The WHO also recommends that a healthy newborn should remain with the mother whenever possible, and that "immediate breast feeding should be encouraged even before the mother leaves the delivery room."[45] But the thirty-six women in the study were only able to see and hold their babies in the recovery room, after delays of several minutes or in one case, more than an hour. The women were kept at the hospital for two nights before being discharged.

Cuba's maternal mortality rate (MMR), the annual number of female deaths per 100,000 live births from any cause related to pregnancy or childbirth, was reported at 77 for 2012, up from 53 in 2008 and 73 in 2010. This is higher than that of many Latin American and Caribbean nations, including Peru (67), Brazil (56), Costa Rica (40), Uruguay (29), and Chile (25), which reported declines in maternal deaths during this period. The aforementioned countries all reported higher infant mortality rates (deaths per 1,000 live births) for 2012 than Cuba's official figure of 4.83: Peru, 21.5; Brazil, 20.5; Costa Rica, 9.2; Uruguay, 9.44; and Chile, 7.36.[46] As levels of maternal and infant mortality usually rise or fall together, this disparity warrants further investigation.

There are disturbing accounts from Cubans living outside the country of pregnant women compelled to have abortions if any fetal anomalies are detected and of very premature infants denied adequate care; their subsequent deaths listed as stillbirths. Such reports are impossible to verify, but what seems certain is that Cuban health professionals are under considerable pressure to adjust their clinical interventions in order to keep the official infant mortality figure low. Katherine Hirschfeld, who conducted research on Cuban health care while residing in the country in the late 1990s, writes that

> Any doctor who had an unusually high rate of infant deaths in his or her jurisdiction would be viewed as having failed in a number of critical respects.
>
> One of the family doctors I worked with in Havana was quite politically militant and took these health goals very seriously. One day during my clinic observations I observed her scheduling an ultrasound for a pregnant woman.
>
> "What happens if an ultrasound shows some fetal abnormalities?" I asked.
>
> "The mother would have an abortion," the doctor replied casually.
>
> "Why?" I queried.

"Otherwise it might raise the infant mortality rate."[47]

Dr. Rodolfo Stusser, a physician and researcher, worked in eastern Cuba in 1972–1974, where he delivered babies as part of his medical practice. He observed the practice of reporting cases of infants born alive but who died in the first minutes after delivery as "intra-partum fetal deaths" as a means to artificially lower the infant mortality rate. He later worked at Havana's Maternity Hospital in 1988 and witnessed that "often living fetuses from induced abortions were thrown alive in the ward bathroom waste basket" and omitted from reports of live births and deaths.

"If these vital events—of at least over twenty-one weeks of gestational age or 499 grams of weight, if not of all ages and weights—would have been reported, Cuba's infant mortality rates would have been at least 50 percent higher," he estimated.[48]

The official figure for low birth weight is just 5 percent, which if true would give Cuba a lower percentage of underweight newborns than France, Germany, and several other Western countries with socialized medicine, according to a comparative list compiled by UNICEF.[49] Blood samples are taken from newborns to screen for Phenylketonuria (PKU) and other conditions and the family doctor is required to make a house call within seventy-two hours of a newborn's arrival from the hospital. There is a series of thirteen vaccinations, and the infant's family receives a kit containing material to be made into diapers. Breastfeeding is encouraged, and according to health ministry officials, half of Cuban infants less than six months old are exclusively breastfed. [50] Young children under seven are supposed to receive a liter of milk as part of their daily rations. Despite these measures, the nutritional status of Cuban babies is uneven: an evaluation of eighty infants less than fourteen months old in three Havana neighborhoods revealed that 72 percent were deficient in iron, 30 percent in calcium, 26 percent in vitamin C, and 31 percent in vitamin A, with smaller deficiencies of other nutrients.[51] Health officials have reported "an absolute predominance" of mild anemia among children under five in Cuba's eastern provinces, and in 2008 the World Food Program and other United Nations agencies began working in Cuba to help produce and distribute iron-fortified foodstuffs.[52]

A child's future health is also affected by living conditions, and Cuba's chronic housing shortage and the deteriorated condition of so many buildings is an obvious negative factor. Water shortages are common in many parts of the country, and 43 percent of rural households and 17 percent of urban households lack running water.[53] In 2011, Cuban authorities revealed that over 100,000 Havana residents were receiving their water via tanker truck, and the National Institute of Water reported that a drought had caused the Cuban capital's water to reach its lowest levels in fifty years.[54] Public service announcements on Cuban television warn viewers to boil water for five minutes before drinking, though water improperly stored in homes can easily become contaminated.

Intestinal ailments and parasitic infections are a common risk to Cuban children, contributing to nutritional deficiencies and if untreated result in a failure to thrive. A sampling of 104 children under five years old at an urban day care center in the city of Matanzas in 2012 revealed that 71.1 percent harbored at least one intestinal parasite and 45.2 percent were infected with more than one species. The researchers cited similar studies of intestinal parasites among preschool children in Brazil and Pakistan, mentioning infection rates lower than those of the Cuban children examined: 29.3 percent and 52.8 percent, respectively (though different sampling techniques might have been used).[55]

A study of schoolchildren, ages six to eleven, in the eastern city of Santiago from 2010 to 2011 showed that 37.8 percent suffered from intestinal parasites and of those children residing in overcrowded households, over three quarters were affected. The study's authors recommended that these results be discussed with "health decision makers in the province, in order to promote healthy habits and lifestyles."[56] Another research study examined blood tests from schoolchildren in western and central Cuba and found that 38.8 percent showed antibodies to *Toxocara canis*, indicating infection with the intestinal roundworms of dogs and that over 50 percent had other parasites such as *Giardia lamblia* and hookworm.[57] A survey of parents, grandparents, and other caregivers at a Havana pediatric hospital revealed awareness of the dangers of intestinal parasites and the importance of hygiene in preventing such infections, yet a number of respondents reported they were not always able to boil their drinking water due to a lack of fuel.[58]

Overcrowded living conditions inevitably increase stress within Cuban households and contribute to another hazard for women and children: domestic violence and sexual abuse. Cuban officials have not published any national figures on violence against women, but a 2007 poll of 250 women between the ages of fifteen and fifty-nine at one Havana polyclinic showed that 55.2 percent had suffered physical violence in their homes, and of those women who had experienced either physical or psychological violence, 71 percent seemed unaware that they were victims of mistreatment.[59]

There are also no published figures on the subject of child sexual abuse and professionals working with Cuban children offer contradictory accounts. According to Michele Frank, an American child and adolescent psychiatrist who studied medicine in Cuba and works in Havana, sex abuse of children within Cuban households is practically nonexistent. When speaking to a group of American visitors, she was asked by a social worker as to how cases of child sex abuse were handled in Cuba. She replied this was something virtually unknown in Cuba, that children were well-cared for and that as neighbors live in close proximity to each other and windows are usually left open, it would be nearly impossible for such acts to be hidden.[60] But Cuban officials have been sufficiently concerned with child sex abuse cases to seek assistance from a British charity, the Child Protection Development Trust, in order to improve investigations into such crimes.

The charity provides specialized video equipment and training in interviewing techniques so that a young victim, rather than being forced to relive the trauma by having to repeat the story on multiple occasions, undergoes a single interview that is recorded and used by police and social service professionals. The Cuban Interior Ministry, having observed the organization's work in Costa Rica, approached the Trust via the British Embassy, and the first child protection center opened in Havana in 2004. Two more centers were subsequently opened in Santiago in 2008 and in Santa Clara in 2011. The centers are located in residential areas, "a deliberate strategy to create a reassuring and friendly environment that did not have the appearance of an official building," with toys and a play area. Prior to the child's visit to the center, background information is collected and the interview is conducted by a plainclothes police officer, briefed by social workers and a psychologist, in a living room with sofas and stuffed animals. Nearly 900 cases were referred to the Havana center during its first two years of operation.[61]

Dr. Tony Butler, a member of the Trust who helped train staff at the centers, said that domestic child sexual abuse in Cuba was a serious issue that followed the same patterns as in many other countries. Cuban officials had not realized the extent of the problem prior to a social survey taken a few years earlier. According to Butler, the Cuban officials he met and worked with over a number of years "took this very seriously as a developing phenomenon in other countries of the region."[62] While he and his colleagues had limited contact with the general population during their visits, they said they sensed a sincere desire on the part of the Cuban officials whom they met to help child sex abuse victims.

The growth of the country's tourism industry has produced concerns that Cuban children could be vulnerable to sexual abuse on the part of foreigners. A report by the Royal Canadian Mounted Police on Canadian child sex abusers describes Cuba as a potential destination for such offenders, noting the country was the second most visited destination among those investigated for traveling child sex offenses. But the report also stated that Cuba, with its high literacy rate, did not have many of the characteristics of other countries frequented by child sex offenders and that "the police and other officials appear to treat sex crimes, particularly those against children, seriously and professionally." Security was good at the larger tourist resorts, but this is not the case at the private homes (*casas particulares*) rented to foreigners, although the owners of such properties are required by law to register such visitors within twenty-four hours of arrival. The report warned that

> Casa particulars, by contrast, allow foreigners to find accommodations in local communities, sometimes in rural areas, for an inexpensive rate. Casa particulars allow foreign travelling child sex offenders to access children and locals who are willing to facilitate crimes against children in return for financial compensation. Poor or dysfunctional families may be particularly willing to open their doors to foreigners with the hope of reaping some financial benefits or so they can receive food or material items. Offenders can, and often do, capitalize on this vulnerability to gain sexual access to child victims.[63]

There have been some well-publicized cases of foreigners abusing Cuban children, such as that of James McTurk, a retired Canadian postal worker twice convicted of child pornography who traveled to Cuba over thirty times over a three-year period prior to his arrest in 2013.[64] North American press coverage of the case, which included a photograph of McTurk holding a picture of Che Guevara, may have prompted Cuban authorities to launch a crackdown on more visible signs of prostitution. A few months later the country's justice minister, Maria Esther Reus, announced that the authorities had prosecuted 224 people for pimping in 2012, that seven foreigners were serving prison sentences in Cuba for sexually abusing children, but that child sex offenses were "minimal." She referred indirectly to the McTurk case and said that cases "such as that of the Canadian are usually used against Cuba politically" and that Cuba's judiciary dealt severely with such crimes. Laritza Diversent, a Cuban lawyer who had worked on prostitution cases, including one involving the death of a twelve-year old girl in 2010, rejected these claims, saying that prostitution was a structural problem in the country and that the government did not want to acknowledge "that a good part of the tourism that reaches Cuba is sex tourism."[65]

Prostitution is not illegal in Cuba, and while Cuban law establishes the age of consent at sixteen, there seems to be little official or unofficial concern over underage sex, even in cases involving predatory adults. An article published in the *Revista Cubana de Pediatria* describes a study of adolescent girls, some just eleven years old, who had sought treatment at a juvenile gynecology clinic in Havana. The young patients, whose ages ranged from eleven to nineteen, were divided into two groups, with one offered informative counseling about contraceptive methods and the other group not. The authors reported that the counseled group demonstrated better contraceptive use, fewer menstrual extractions, and a better cure rate for cervicitis and vaginal infections.[66]

The Hogar Materno Leonor Perez, located in Havana's historic district, is a showcase maternity home and a frequent stop on many foreign delegations' tours of Cuba. A group of American visitors asked the ages of the oldest and youngest pregnant woman who had stayed at the home. The oldest mother, a doctor told the group, was in her fifties and the youngest, just twelve, impregnated by a forty-nine-year-old man. Was he prosecuted, the visitors wanted to know. No, the doctor said, for the girl's family did not bring charges and it was the man's first child.[67]

NOTES

1. "State of the World's Mothers 2013," Save the Children, http://www.savethechildren.org/atf/cf/%7B9def2ebe-10ae-432c-9bd0-df91d2eba74a%7D/SOWM-FULL-REPORT_2013.PDF.
2. World Bank figures.
3. Sergio Diaz-Briquets and Lisandro Perez,"Fertility Decline in Cuba: A Socioeconomic Interpretation," *Population and Development Review*, Vol. 8, No. 3 (September 1982), pp. 513–537. The authors cite figures showing Cuba's fertility rate was lower than Canada's and about the same as that of the United States, Australia, New Zealand, and Portugal.
4. The official figure is 4.76 per thousand live births, and 5.90 in the United States, according to the CIA World Factbook.
5. Yasmany Diaz of CENESEX spoke to a Global Exchange tour group, which included the author, on November 15, 2012.
6. Bertha Gonzalez Valcarcel, Elsa Núñez Aragón, Lourdes Couturejuzon González, and Zoraida Amable Ambrós, "Conocimientos y comportamientos sobre el VIH/SIDA en adolescentes de enseñanza media superior," *Revista Cubana Salud Publica*, Vol. 34 No. 2 (April–June 2008).
7. Jorge Alejandro Rodriquez, "¿Qué sucede con los condones?" *Juventud Rebelde*, January 1, 2013.
8. Leslie Diaz Monserrat, "Ausencias peligrosas," *Vanguardia*, April 3, 2014.
9. Leslie Diaz Monserrat, "Mas sobre la venta de condones," *Vanguardia*, April 18, 2014. See also Juan O. Tamayo, "Cuba moves to end condom shortage by selling stock with the 'wrong expiration dates,'" *Miami Herald*, April 20, 2014.
10. Braulio Heredia Hernandez, Evelio L. Cabezas Cruz, Alejandro Velazco Boza, and Raoul Gazapo Pernas, "Una nueva opción anticonceptiva noristerat inyectable," *Revista Cubana de Obstetricia y Ginecologia*, June 1996.
11. Armando Seuc Jo, Felipe Santana Perez, Roberto M. Gonzalez Suarez, Maria Celeste Arranz Calzado, and Gloria M. Fernandez Lopez, "Efecto del contraceptivo inyectable Depo-Provera sobre el metabolismo de la glucosa," *Revista Cubana Endocrinol*, Vol. 11, No. 2 (2000), pp. 98–104.
12. Statement by the Cuban delegation at the 44th Session of the Commission on Population and Development, under agenda item 4: "General debate on national experience in population matters: fertility, reproductive health and development," http://www.un.org/en/development/desa/population/pdf/commission/2011/country/agendaitem4/cuba.pdf
13. Diaz-Briquets and Perez, op. cit., footnote 10.
14. Danièle Bélanger and Andrea Flynn, "The Persistence of Induced Abortion in Cuba: Exploring the Notion of an "Abortion Culture," *Studies in Family Planning*, March 2009, pp. 13–26.
15. Ibid.
16. British Broadcasting Corporation, February 25, 1998.
17. Elías Biscet González and Rolando Muñoz Yyobre, "El Rivanol: un método para destruir la vida," *Lawton Foundation*. April 1998.
18. United Nations data, http://data.un.org/Data.aspx?d=GenderStat&f=inID%3A12. Accessed on June 7, 2013.
19. Maria Gran, "Interrupcion voluntaria de embarazo y anticoncepción: Dos metodos de regulacion de la fecundidad. Cuba. 1995–2000," City of Havana, 2004.
20. Bélanger and Flynn, op. cit.
21. Interview with Dr. Alberto Dominguez-Bali, August 23, 2013.

22. Alfonso de Armas, Marisol, "Family planning and reproductive and sexual health in Cuba," *Asociación Latinoamericana de Población*, http://www.alapop.org/docs/publicaciones/investigaciones/DemogTransformations_ParteIII-5.pdf

23. Lainelys, Abreu, "Un método quirúrgico a ciegas," *Somos Jovenes* digital edition, July 24–31, 2013. Accessed July 27, 2013.

24. These include an iron supplement and a multivitamin, Prenatal. While ordinarily these would be given as soon as pregnancy is diagnosed (or before, if a woman is trying to conceive), many women do not receive these supplements until the second trimester, according to an investigation by the digital newspaper Cafe Fuerte, http://cafefuerte.com/cuba/noticias-de-cuba/sociedad/2841-cuanto-cuesta-tener-un-hijo-en-cuba.

25. Text of speech by Fidel Castro, April 7, 2003, http://www.granma.cu/documento/ingles03/013.html.

26. "Cuban Health Care: "Aquí Nada es Facil (Nothing is Easy)," confidential cable from the U.S. Interests Section in Havana, dated January 31, 2008, http://www.cablegatesearch.net/cable.php?id=08HAVANA103&q=cuba.

27. "Maternity Waiting Homes: A Review of Experiences," World Health Organization, 1996, http://whqlibdoc.who.int/hq/1996/WHO_RHT_MSM_96.21.pdf.

28. Ibid.

29. Oficina Nacional de Estadisticas (ONE), figures for 2011.

30. Gisela Pita Rodriguez et al, "Ingesta de macronutrientes y vitaminas en embarazadas durante un año," *Revista Cubana Salud Pública*, Vol. 29, No. 3 (2003), pp. 220–227.

31. "Apoyo a la lucha contra la anemia en grupos vulnerables en Cuba," United Nations Development Program, September 2009.

32. Elise Andaya, "Conceiving Statistics: The Local Practice and Politics of Reproductive Health Care in Havana," in *Health Travels: Cuban Health(care) On and Off the Island*, Nancy Burke, ed (San Francisco: University of California Medical Humanities Consortium, 2013).

33. Manuel Franco, Usama Bilal, Pedro Benet Orduñez, Alain Mikhail Morejon, Joan Kennely, and Richard Cooper, "Population-wide weight loss and regain in relation to diabetes burden and cardiovascular mortality in Cuba 1980–2010: Repeated cross sectional surveys and ecological comparison of secular trends," *British Medical Journal*, April 9, 2013.

34. Feinsilver, op. cit., p. 73.

35. Carmen Porrata, "Cubans' Deadly Diet: A Wakeup Call," *MEDICC Review*, Vol. 10, No. 2 (Spring 2008).

36. "One more number in the statistics," with photo of the prescribed diet (*consulta de nutricion*), dated May 16, 2011 and posted May 21, 2011, http://octavocercoen.blogspot.co.uk/2011/05/breakfast-1-c.html.

37. Cited in Patricia Varona, Marcha Chang, Rene Garcia, and Mariano Bonet, "Tobacco and Alcohol Use in Cuban Women," *MEDICC Review*, Vol. 13, No. 4 (October 2011)

38. Nery Suárez Lugo, Magali Caraballoso Hernández, and Sandra Hechavarria Negrín, "El tabaquismo en los profesionales de la salud en el municipio Habana Vieja," *Revista Cubana Salud Publica*, Vol. 34, No. 4 (October–December 2008).

39. According to *MEDICC Review*, Vol. 7, No. 6 (June 2005): "fathers have been permitted in the *labor* (emphasis added) room in every maternity hospital in Cuba" since February 2005. The same MEDICC article also states, incorrectly, that this is "currently not an option in most health institutions worldwide," http://www.medicc.org/publications/medicc_review/0605/headlines-in-cuban-health.html. Another article in the same issue states that "Men do, however, increasingly attend the birth of their children," http://www.medicc.org/publications/medicc_review/0605/mr-features.html. In fact, Cuba is one of the few countries in the world where fathers are not allowed to be present during the birth of their children. A physician at the Leonor Perez maternity home in Havana told the author's tour group on November 14, 2012 that fathers were not allowed in the delivery room. Stephanie Bernal, the author of

"Women's Health Care in Cuba: Observation of Medical Facilities in Cerro, Havana," received two different explanations for this: "According to Dr. Sosa-Leyva, the presence of men in the delivery room might make the delivery too chaotic (personal communication, June 27, 2000). A more experienced doctor whose specializes in obstetrics noted that the small delivery room makes it impossible to allow the father to attend the birth (J. Puentes-Corral, personal communication, July 6, 2000)." *International Perspectives, the Journal of California State University, San Bernadino's International Institute,* Vol. 1 (Spring 2001).

40. Dailys Garcia-Jorda, Zoe Diaz-Bernal, and Marlen Acosta Alamo, "El nacimiento en Cuba: análisis de la experiencia del parto medicalizado desde una perspectiva antropológica," *Ciencia y Saude Coletiva,* Vol. 17, No. 7 (June 2012). Rio de Janeiro, Brazil

41. Beverly Chalmers, "WHO appropriate technology for birth revisited," *British Journal of Obstetrics and Gynaecology,* Vol. 99 (September 1992), pp. 709–710.

42. Garcia-Jorda, op. cit.

43. Chalmers, op. cit.

44. Garcia-Jorda, op. cit.

45. Chalmers, op. cit.

46. CIA World Factbook.

47. Katherine Hirschfeld, "Re-examing the Cuban Health Care System: Towards a Qualitative Critique," *Cuban Affairs,* Vol. 2, Issue 3 (July 2007).

48. Stusser, Rodolfo J., "Demystifying the Cuban Health System: An Insider's View," paper presented to the Association for the Study of the Cuban Economy(ASCE) conference, Miami 2011.

49. http://www.childinfo.org/low_birthweight_profiles.php.

50. Statement made by Dr. Pablo Roque Peña, coordinator of the Ministry of Public Health's breast feeding program, "one of every two infants less than six months of age are exclusively breastfed." Quoted in Israel Hernandez Alvarez, "More infants exclusively breastfed in Cuba," *Granma,* August 9, 2013.

51. Mayleni Carrillo Selles, Onay Mercader Camejo, Gisela Pita Rodriguez, "Evaluación dietética de micronutrientes en niños entre 10 y 14 meses de edad," *Revista Cubana de Pediatria,* Vol. 80 No. 4 (October–December 2008).

52. Lisett Nancy Selva Suárez and Alcides Abad Ochoa Alonso, "Acciones para la prevención y control de la anemia por deficiencia de hierro en niños hasta cinco años," *Revista Cubana de Salud Pública,* Vol. 3 (2011).

53. "Cuba: estimates of the use of water sources and sanitation facilities (1980-2011)," WHO/UNICEF Joint Monitoring Program (JMP) for Water Supply and Sanitation, http://www.wssinfo.org/documents-links/documents/?tx_displaycontroller%5Btype%5D=country_files.

54. *Granma,* April 12, 2011.

55. Roberto Cañete, Manuska Morales Diaz, Roxana Avalos Garcia, Pedro Miguel Laúd Martinez, and Felix Manuel Ponce, "Intestinal Parasites from a Day Care Center in Matanzas City Cuba," http://www.plosone.org/article/info%3Adoi%2F10.1371%2Fjournal.pone.0051394

56. Glenda Perez Sanchez et al, "Prevalencia de parasitismo intestinal en escolares de 6-11 años," *MEDISAN,* Vol. 16, No. 4 (April 2012). http://scielo.sld.cu/scielo.php?script=sci_arttext&pid=S1029-30192012000400009. By way of comparison, Cuban physicians working in Ecuatorial Guinea conducted research into parasitic infection among schoolchildren in that country, and found a significantly lower level of infection—29.9 percent—than what has been reported among Cuban children. See "Parasitismo intestinal en una escuela primaria de Bata, Guinea Ecuatorial," *Revista Ciencias Medicas,* Vol. 12, No. 1 (April 2008), http://scielo.sld.cu/scielo.php?pid=S1561-31942008000100008&script=sci_arttext.

57. K. Kanobana Sariego, R. Junco, K. Vereecken, F. A. Nunez, K. Polman, M. Bonet, and L. Rojas, "Frequency of antibodies to *Toxocara* in Cuban schoolchildren," *Tropical Medicine and International Health,* Vol. 17, No. 6 (June 2012), pp. 711–714.

58. Angel A. Escobedo, Pedro Almirall, Maydel Alfonso, Ivonne Avila, Sergio Cimermana, Yohana Salazar, Isabel V. Dawkins, and Rosa M. Garcia, "Caregiver perspectives for the prevention, diagnosis and treatment of childhood giardiasis in Havana City, Cuba: A qualitative study," *Acta Tropica*, Vol. 119, Issues 2–3 (August 2011), pp. 99–106.

59. Odalys Gil Lopez, "Situación de la violencia doméstica en la mujer, en la población del policlínico 'Julio Antonio Mella,'" *Revista Cubana de Medicina Integral General*, Vol. 27 No. 4 (Oct–Dec 2011).

60. Remarks made Dr. Michele Frank in Havana on Saturday, November 17, 2012 to a Global Exchange tour group in which the author participated.

61. Child Protection Development Trust, http://cpdtrust.org/en/project-cuba-1.htm

62. Interview with Tony Butler, June 11, 2012.

63. Michael Serapiglia and Melanie Laroche, "Project SUNRISE: Targeting Canadian Travelling Child Sex Offenders," http://media.elnuevoherald.com/smedia/2013/03/13/10/50/a3cPA.So.84.pdf.

64. "James McTurk: Portrait of an alleged sex tourist in Cuba," *Miami Herald*, March 16, 2013.

65. "Cuba's Justice Minister says the government fights prostitution," *Miami Herald*, October 16, 2013.

66. Miguel Lugones Botell, Marieta Ramírez Bermúdez, Hector Machado Rodriguez, "Intervención educativa en adolescentes atendidas en consulta de ginecología infanto-juvenil," *Revista Cubana de Pediatria*, Vol. 80, No. 2 (April–June 2008).

67. Comments made during author's tour group visit to the Hogar Materno Leonor Perez in Havana, November 14, 2012.

FOUR

Aging and Youth: A Cuban Dilemma

The elderly newspaper vendor was painfully thin, walking slowly and with difficulty as he made his way along the pavement outside Havana's Museum of the Revolution. He carried only a few copies of *Granma*, the official organ of the Cuban Communist Party, which he tried to sell to foreigners boarding a tourist bus. The same tour group would be taken later to one of Cuba's showcase facilities for the elderly, the Convento de Belen senior center, which their itinerary had erroneously listed as being run by the Catholic Church. Upon arrival, the group was briskly informed by a matron that the center was operated by the Cuban government, not the church, and guided to a seating area where a comedy skit about bus riders was about to begin. Outside the building, more elderly Cub ans were assembling for a morning exercise class.[1]

The Convento de Belen, a restored eighteenth-century building in Havana's historic district, offers the elderly arts and crafts workshops, social activities, and has a pharmacy, physical therapy, and ophthalmology/optometrist units. The approximately 600 elderly Havana residents who use the center's services each day are probably more fortunate than many older Cubans, for while retirement is not mandatory in Cuba, it is also a luxury that many of the country's older citizens cannot afford. Fidel and Raul Castro's generation witnessed the Revolution and now finds itself waiting for basic resources and services amid continuing shortages and a shrinking base of working adults to provide these goods and services.

A 2004 survey of 164 elderly Cubans in Pinar del Rio revealed that 56.2 percent were still working, with 80 percent of men in urban areas and 85 percent of men in rural areas still employed.[2] Another study in the same province polled 80 elderly people who lived at home with their families and asked them to rate their household relationships as very harmonic, harmonic, unharmonic, or very unharmonic. A majority (71.4

percent) of those still employed described their family interactions as either very harmonic (*"muy armonicas"*) or harmonic, while of those elderly Cubans who were not working, 79.1 percent rated their relationships as either unharmonic or very unharmonic.[3]

There are no published figures on the number of older Cubans whom economic necessity has pushed into the country's informal economy, but elderly vendors selling newspapers, candy, and other goods are a common sight in urban areas. Cuban state salaries are meager, and pensions are even more so, and a typical retiree's income might range from $8–12 per month, barely enough to cover a week's worth of food. Many needed medicines and medical supplies can only be found on the black market. For those Cubans without support from relatives abroad, or access to convertible pesos, day-to-day existence can be very harsh.

Cuba's population is aging rapidly, as a result of low birth rates and high emigration rates, especially among adults of working age. The chart below shows Cuba's population by age range, based on the 2012 national census.[4]

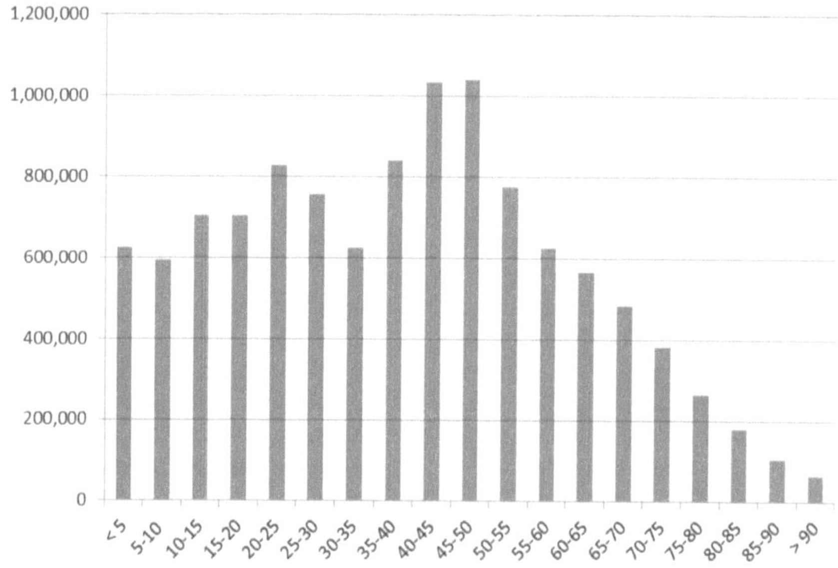

Figure 4.1.

Life expectancy has reached seventy-six years for men and eighty for women, with an increasing number of Cubans living into their eighties and longer. According to the University of Havana's Center for Demographic Studies (CEDEM), if current trends continue, well over a quarter of the Cuban population will be over sixty in 2025 and by 2050 this figure will reach 34 percent.[5] Low birth rates and high emigration rates are largely to blame: the number of Cubans leaving their country has increased steadily over the past two decades and many of those emigrants are among those with the most drive and ambition. In 1980 over 140,000 Cubans left the country when authorities announced that anyone wanting to leave could do so freely; approximately 125,000 arrived in the United States. Another, less massive exodus occurred in 1994 when nearly 48,000 were allowed to leave, many boarding flimsy rafts heading toward Florida. The Castro government then reimposed travel restrictions and three years later the number of emigrants had dropped to 21,000 and then began to increase again, reaching 46,662 in 2012, according to Cuba's National Statistics Office.[6] In January 2013, Cuban authorities liberalized travel restrictions, allowing more people to leave the country legally and to return without suffering any confiscation of property within twenty-four months, and with a provision allowing an extension of another twenty-four months. The measure prompted a 35 percent increase in Cubans traveling during the first ten months of the year, and while the new policy seemed designed to stem the population loss, only 57.8 percent returned after leaving the country, according to the Dirección de Inmigración y Extranjería.[7]

The pressure of a declining workforce supporting an increasing proportion of the population that is aging cannot be sustained indefinitely. While this is a significant issue in many countries, Cuba is especially affected by an already shaky economic base. The retirement age had historically been sixty years for men, fifty-five for women but in recent years officials moved to raise this requirement with a phased program. Starting in 2009, the retirement age was increased by six months every year, culminating in 2018 when Cuba was expected to have a retirement age of sixty-five for men and sixty for women. Those continuing to work past retirement age have grown at twice the rate of the overall workforce, the result of greater need and some government incentives. After thirty years of service, a retiree will receive a pension equal to 90 percent of his or her salary, with an extra 2 percent earned for every additional year of work. Those in technical, educational, or other professional fields also have the option to work and add salary to their pension.[8]

Changing demographics have altered the composition of households in Cuba. The decline in the fertility rate has caused the average number of individuals per household to drop from 4.9 to 3.2 over the last fifty years. The makeup of these households has evolved over time as well so that 54 percent of households are traditional nuclear families while 32 percent include members of the extended family. So while nuclear families are dropping in size, extended family households are becoming larger and the average age of these extended family households has been increasing over time as well, with 70 percent of multigenerational homes headed by someone sixty-five or older.[9]

The Cuban capital has a higher percentage of older residents—19.5 percent—than the national average but in the view of architect and urban planner Miguel Coyula, Havana is "no city for old people." From a perspective of equity and social inclusion, Havana's services and infrastructure are inadequate and "are still more inadequate for older adults." In the capital's central municipalities, 85 percent of the housing stock is over eighty years old, usually with architectural barriers such as "stairs-only entrances, without washroom facilities designed for older or disabled persons, limiting their access and contributing to social isolation."[10] Shortages of wheelchairs, walkers, and other assistive devices, combined with the crumbling condition of city sidewalks and streets add to this seclusion.

A survey was published in 2001 of 144 elderly Havana residents with no signs of dementia who lived with their spouses or partners in multigenerational households. It revealed "a predominance of little harmonic or non-harmonic relations, difficulties in defining the inter-generation limits, rigid family hierarchical structure and intolerant attitudes toward the characteristics and behaviors of the elderly people on the part of their families." Nearly half of those surveyed showed signs of moderate to severe depression, and the study's authors noted the obvious link between family relationships and an elderly person's emotional and physical well-being.[11]

Economic hardship causes health indicators to deteriorate, and shortages and scarcity during the "special period in time of peace," following the collapse of the Soviet Union hit elderly Cubans especially hard, with food rations reduced for all but young children and pregnant women. Calorie intake dropped from a daily average of 2,899 per capita in 1988 to 1,940, or a 32 percent decrease, caused by a drop in imports combined by reduced agricultural production as supplies of fertilizer and other products diminished. Dietary fat and animal protein were reduced, while simple carbohydrates increased from 64 percent of the average Cuban's diet in 1990 to 79.4 percent in 1993, with most of this intake a combination of polished white rice and refined cereal, affecting critical amino acid intake. Poor nutrition and the added stresses also increased mortality rates associated with noncommunicable diseases among the elderly. The rate of death for those aged sixty-five or over increased by more than 10 percent for each of the following: cardiac disease, diarrheal disease, influenza, pneumonia, and tuberculosis.[12] Mortality rates associated with heart disease were brought back under control in the latter part of the decade, but disease processes associated with failing infrastructure—food supplies, housing, water, and sewage—were not mitigated.

One unintended benefit of this period was an increase in physical activity, as fuel shortages forced Cubans to walk or bicycle more. Between 1987 and 1995, those leading a sedentary lifestyle were reduced from 62 percent to 25.7 percent for men and from 78 percent to 39.8 percent for women. Walking increased by 22 percent for men and 26.1 percent for women, and those who rode bicycles increased by 47.1 percent for men and 17.4 percent for women.

Partly as a result of this increased physical activity, those who were overweight dropped by 41 percent for women and 52.4 percent for men and the rate of obesity dropped by 43 percent for women and 61 percent for men. But by 1996 food was becoming more available and caloric intake began to increase, reaching a daily average of 2,335 per capita, with both vegetable and fat intake increased. By 1996, those in Havana who had been overweight regained much of this lost weight, with 43 percent of women and 49 percent of men now overweight and obesity levels grew by a significant 64 percent for women and 61 percent for men.

This yo-yo weight loss and regain produced a number of disturbing trends. From 1988 to 1998 the incidence of hypertension increased from 4.9 percent of the population to nearly 13 percent. The rate of diabetes mellitus grew from 16.5 to 21.5 per 1,000 inhabitants during this period. Women aged sixty to sixty-four were especially affected, with the rate increasing from 70.4 per 1,000 to 122 per 1,000. Colon and rectal cancer also increased during this period and the resulting mortality rates increased as well.

At the end of the decade, one study found that a majority of older Havana residents were either overweight or underweight. Researchers examined the body mass index of 1,905 people aged sixty and over, and found that 33 percent were underweight and those overweight were 29.6 percent, with those eighty and over less likely to be overweight. "The elderly population of Havana presents a vulnerable nutritional status in view of the prevalence of underweight and overweight increasing age, smoking, gender and hypertension are the factors positively associated with vulnerable nutritional status," the study concluded.[13]

There have been a number of government programs over the years aimed at improving the welfare of Cubans entering the "third age." In 1974, officials implemented the Elder Care National Plan, which was modified several years later following recommendations from a U.N. World Assembly on Aging held in Vienna. The Assembly listed the following objectives (along with 62 scientific recommendations):[14]

a. The economic, social and cultural implication of aging is to be understood within countries, as well as globally, to support the aging of populations.
b. Humanitarian and developmental issues relating to aging are to be understood both nationally and globally.
c. Policies and programs that may be implemented to insure social and financial security for the aged should be promoted. In addition, the intent is to allow the elderly to be involved in contributing to, and share the benefits of a country's development.
d. Options for programmatic and policy implementation consistent with national standards as they relate to the aging of the population are to be proposed.

e. The development of appropriate education and training programs as well as a research agenda to meet the needs of a global aging population is to be promoted. There should be sharing of ideas globally.

It is not clear how the recommendations affected the welfare of Cuba's elderly, but the family doctor and nurse program begun in 1984 should have resulted in better coordinated services for this age group. The following year, the University of Havana's Center for Demographic Studies undertook an extensive study on the health and social circumstances of older Cubans, partly funded by the United Nations, the University of Montreal, and Duke University.

The report said Cuba had fulfilled the Vienna Plan's recommendations on income security and social assistance, and that the percentage of elderly Cubans still forced to work had decreased from 40.7 percent in 1953 to 17.2 percent in 1970, with further decreases forecast for the future. The majority of Cubans over sixty—69.5 percent—were suffering from chronic diseases such as heart disease, hypertension, diabetes, and asthma and 16 percent were reported to have vision problems ranging from "bad" to blindness. 80.7 percent reported their hearing as either "good" or "very good." Nearly half (49.7 percent) were missing all their teeth while 44.7 percent were missing some or most of their teeth. The report says nothing about the availability of dentures during this period, but warns that "dental failure might lead to poor nutrition." Just over half had corns, calluses, and bunions on their feet which made it difficult to walk, and 47.9 percent had "poor performance of the arms and feet."[15]

In 1996 Cuba unveiled another plan to help the country's elderly, the "Integral Program of Attention to the Older Adult," which sought to expand social and medical services. Two years later authorities began forming teams of eldercare specialists, comprised og a physician, a nurse, a psychologist, and a social worker with a diploma in gerontology and geriatrics and by 2005 there were 436 such teams in the country.[16] Social groups for elderly Cubans, *Circulos de Abuelos*, or grandparents' circles, were formed in local polyclinics around the country to promote social interaction, exercise, and physical and mental health, which involved a relatively small investment of public funds. There is also a network of *Casas de Abuelos*, over 200 elder day care centers which offer social and cultural activities, along with some level of services from a nurse or social workers and are generally open eight to ten hours on weekdays. There are also 127 residential care homes for the elderly throughout the country. But even Cuban officials admit that the available resources do not meet the needs of the country's aging population. The senior day centers and residential facilities also suffer from the same deteriorated conditions found in so many other Cuban health facilities. At a care home in Cienfuegos, residents complained that the facility only had water on alternate days, and then only for three hours at a time.[17] There have also been numerous reports of employees stealing soap, detergent, and other supplies at the homes, and of outbreaks of scabies and other infections caused by poor hygiene.[18] According to an account by an independent Cuban news site, a refrigerator, a television set, and two air conditioners had been purloined by staff members at the Hogar de Ancianos Chung Wah in Havana, and quickly returned when health officials announced an inspection of the facility.[19]

The Catholic Church has been allowed to provide some services to the elderly and other vulnerable groups and operates homes for the elderly in Havana and Camaguey, which are reported to be so well-regarded that there are unofficial waiting lists.[20] Caritas, the Catholic charity, reports that "undernourishment is a chronic problem on the island,"[21] and has about 400 projects around the country, including 190 canteens providing meals for 28,000 elderly people. A volunteer at one of the centers in Matanzas province said food was prepared three times a week, and that many take their meals home to ration it over a couple of days or else share it with another household member. The charity also takes food to elderly housebound Cubans.[22] Nevertheless, some of the elderly participants in the program have been interrogated by Cuban police.[23]

Alberto Fernandez Seco, head of MINSAP's Older Adults, Social Assistance and Mental Health Department, gave an interview to the official government newspaper *Granma* in which he said that requests for places in Cuba's care homes were greater than the existing capacity nationwide. The day centers can accommodate 7,398 people, though demand is estimated at over 20,000 and the country's nursing homes have only 9,287 beds. He said Cuba's health system, which historically had emphasized maternal-infant care or "illnesses of short duration which do not result in disability," now needed to train more geriatric specialists. At present, he said, there were only 279 such physicians working in the country and another 137 undergoing training.[24] There is likely to be an even greater demand for nurses to care for aging patients. Cuba's nurse ratio is 90 per 10,000 population, well above that of most developing countries but lower than that of the United States, Canada, and many European countries, all of which have nursing shortages but whose elder population is proportionately smaller than Cuba's.[25]

Increasing numbers of Cubans will suffer from Alzheimer's and dementia, and according to Juan Llibre, who chaired the fifth Ibero American conference on the disease in Havana in 2011, the country already has 130,000 such cases. This figure could reach 300,000 in 2040 if current trends continue, he said.[26] Cuba also has higher dementia prevalence rates compared with other Caribbean countries in the same geographic area, and some researchers have speculated that chronic nutritional deficiencies during the special period and beyond could be a factor.

There was an epidemic of optic and peripheral neuropathy causing impaired vision and numbness, caused by vitamin B deficiency, with those ages forty-five to sixty-four among the most affected.[27] The first cases were reported in November of 1991, when eight middle-aged men in the western province of Pinar del Rio experienced a loss of vision. By July of the following year there were 168 such cases. On August 22 prison inmates in Cienfuegos on the southern coast of Cuba were hospitalized with edema, difficulty walking, and weakness, all preceded by weight loss. New cases continued to appear, with some patients reporting hearing loss as well as other symptoms and in March of 1993 the Castro government organized a national task force to study and treat the epidemic, which affected over 50,000 people. Health investigators looked for possible neurotoxins, but the real culprit was poor nutrition and patients were treated with vitamin supplements.[28]

Nutritional deficiencies have persisted into the twenty-first century, especially among older adults. A study by researchers from Cuba's Instituto de Nutrición e Higiene de los Alimentos examined levels of the B1 and B2 vitamin in a sample of fifty noninstitutionalized adults aged sixty and over in two *areas de salud* in Havana. The researchers found that 65 percent were lacking in B1 and 64 percent lacking in B2, indicating a continuing problem with ensuring adequate nutrition among older Cubans.[29]

Cancer and heart disease are the leading causes of death in Cuba, followed by cerebrovascular diseases, influenza, pneumonia, accidents, respiratory diseases, circulatory diseases, diabetes, and "intentional self-harm," or suicide.[30] Cuba's suicide rate of 12.3 per inhabitants per year is the highest in Latin America, and is highest among those sixty and older, followed by those aged forty to fifty-nine. [31]

NOTES

1. Author's observations during a visit to the Convento de Belen senior center in Havana, November 14, 2012.
2. Omaida Rosa Hernández Jiménez, Dr. Manolo Gómez Juanola, and Dra. Mayra Moya Rodríguez, "Caracterización socioeconómica de los ancianos pertenecientes a 2 consultorios médicos del policlínico San Diego de los Baños," *Revista Cubana de Enfermeria*, Vol 22, No. 1 (January–March 2006).
3. Dr. Manolo Gómez Juanola, Albanis Lopez Zamora, Omaida Rosa Hernández Jiménez, and Dra. Mayra Moya Rodriguez, "Influencia de algunas variables en las relaciones familiares del adulto mayor," *Revista Cubana de Medicina General Integral*, Vol. 21, Nos. 1–2 (2005).
4. Oficina Nacional de Estadistica e Informacion, Censo de Población y Viviendas 2012, "Cuba: Viviendas Ocupadas con Residentes Permanentes por Indicadores Seleccionados," http://www.one.cu/publicaciones/cepde/cpv2012/20140428informenacional/29_grafico_19_20.pdf.
5. Rolando Garcia-Quinones, "Social policies, family arrangements and population ageing in Cuba," United Nations Population Fund UNFPA, June 2009.

6. Anuario Demográfico de Cuba 2012, Oficina Nacional de Estadistica e Informacion, http://www.onei.cu/publicaciones/cepde/anuario_2012/12_anuario_MIGRACIONES.pd.
7. "Los viajes de Cubanos de la Isla aumentaron un 35 por ciento," *Cubanet*, October 29, 2013, http://www.cubanet.org/actualidad/los-viajes-de-cubanos-de-la-isla-aumentaron-un35-por-ciento-desde-reforma-migratoria/
8. Patricia Grogg, "Cuba A Good Old Age in Havana," *Inter Press Service*, March 5, 2010; and Garcia-Quinones, op. cit.
9. Garcia-Quinones, op. cit.
10. Miguel Coyula, "Havana: Aging in an Aging City," *MEDICC Review*, Vol. 12, No. 4 (October 2010).
11. Tamara B. Domínguez González, Ana Margarita Espín Andrade, and Héctor Bayorre Vea, "Caracterization de las relaciones familiares del anciano," *Revista Cubana de Medicina General Integral*, Vol. 17, No. 5 (2001), pp. 418–422.
12. A. Rodríguez-Ojea, S. Jiménez, A. Berdasco, and M. Esquivel, "The nutrition transition in Cuba in the nineties: an overview," *Public Health Nutrition* 5.1A (2002), pp. 129–133.
13. , R. Da Silva Coqueiro, A. Rodriguez Barrosa, and A. Ferreti Borgatto, "Nutritional status, health conditions and socio-demographic factors in the elderly of Havana, Cuba: data from SABE survey," *The Journal of Nutrition, Health and Aging*, October 2012.
14. Vienna International Plan of Action on Aging, World Assembly on Aging, July 26-August 6, 1982, Vienna. Austria. http://www.un.org/es/globalissues/ageing/docs/vipaa.pdf
15. Rafael Hernandez Castellon, "Population Ageing in Cuba," Center for Demographic Studies, University of Havana, 1994.
16. Yuselys Malegon Cruz, Adialys Guevara Gonzalez, and Ludmilla Brenes Hernandez, "El envejecimiento demográfico y la atención al Adulto Mayor en Cuba," *GEROINFO*, RNPS, 2110, Vol. 2, No. 2 (2007), http://www.sld.cu/galerias/pdf/sitios/gericuba/envejecimiento_demografico.pdf.
17. Félix Reyes Gutiérrez, "Hogar de ancianos sin agua en Cienfuegos," *Cubanet*, July 25, 2012, http://www.cubanet.org/noticias/hogar-de-ancianos-sin-agua-en-cienfuegos/.
18. Reinaldo Emilio Cosano Alen, "Chung Wah, un dantesco almacén de ancianos," *Cubanet*, December 14, 2012, http://www.cubanet.org/articulos/chung-wah-un-dantesco-almacen-de-ancianos/; and "Brote de escabiosis en hogar de ancianos," *Cubanet*, January 24, 2013, http://www.cubanet.org/noticias/brote-de-escabiosis-en-hogar-de-ancianos/.
19. Reinaldo Emilio Cosano Alen, "Devuelven electrodomésticos a un asilo de ancianos," *Cubanet*, February 14, 2013, http://www.cubanet.org/noticias/devuelven-electrodomesticos-a-un-asilo-de-ancianos/.
20. Tamayo, Juan, "Cuba's Catholic Church trying to fill gaps in social safety net," *Miami Herald*, March 14, 2012.
21. From the Caritas Cuba page, http://crs.org/countries/cuba.
22. Caritas International, "Caritas Cuba helps elderly as poverty grows," March 21, 2012, http://www.caritas.org/2012/03/caritas-cuba-helps-elderly-as-poverty-grows/.
23. Damien Cave, "Some Who Fled Cuba Are Returning to Help," *New York Times*, March 4, 2014.
24. *Granma*, November 21, 2013.
25. "Global Health Facts," The Henry J. Kaiser Family Foundation, http://kff.org/global-indicator/nurses-and-midwives.
26. "El regimen alerta sobre increment del Alzheimer," *Cubanet*, September 20, 2012.
27. Yeneisy Lanya Dominguez, Manuel Hernandez, Consuelo Macias Matos, and Dequan Zhou, "Is B Vitamins Deficiency Associated with Prevalence of Alzheimer's Disease in Cuban Elderly?" *Nutrition and Health*, Vol. 18 (2006), pp. 101–118.

28. Gustavo C. Román, "An epidemic in Cuba of optic neuropathy, sensorineural deafness,peripheral sensory neuropathy and dorsolateral myeloneuropathy," *Journal of the Neurological Sciences*, Vol. 127 (1994), pp. 11–28.

29. Yeneisy Lanyau, Daimí Pineda, Manuel Hernández, Isabel Martín, Maria E. Díaz, and Emilia Toledo, "Estado nutricional y vitaminas B1 y B2 en ancianos no institucionalizados," *Revista Cubana de Salud Publica*, Vol. 29, No. 3 (2003), pp. 209–14.

30. Pan American Health Organization figures.

31. World Health Organization figures, http://www.who.int/mental_health/media/cuba.pdf.

FIVE

Cuban Medical Training

The University of Havana, founded in 1728, is one of the oldest universities in the Americas and contains what for centuries was Cuba's only medical school. The *Facultad de Medicina* was one of the institution's five original departments and prior to the Revolution admitted between 800 and 1,000 students per year, with an average graduation rate of 375 students per year.[1] High school graduates seeking admission were first required to spend a year in a premedical program, studying biology, chemistry, physics, pathology, and one foreign language. Upon successful completion of this premedical program those admitted to the medical school then embarked on a program of study which seemed at least as rigorous as that of medical schools in industrialized countries. Cuban medical students spent the first two years taking courses in anatomy, physiology, histology, embryology, pharmacology, and biochemistry. A further two years of medical study included additional coursework in anatomy as well as pathology, parasitology and tropical diseases, radiology, and obstetrics, followed by two years of clinical studies, as explained in 1930 by the school's director, Dr. I. F. Rodriguez Molina, who observed that "all Cubans want to be lawyers or doctors":

> In these two years they need to complete the medical clinic, two years; surgical clinic, two years; clinical pathology, two years; gynecology, one year; diseases of children, one year; genito-urinary diseases, seventy-five lectures; orthopaedics, seventy-five lectures; diseases of the eye and diseases of the ear, nose and throat, each thirty lectures; and thirty to forty-five practical courses in small groups. We have another year of dermatological diseases and syphilis; mental diseases, thirty-five lectures; hygiene and legal medicine.
>
> When they have finished all this material, they are required to stand an examination. These examinations are in two parts, one of which is clinical. In this clinical work they have to demonstrate before the exam-

> iners one case of children's diseases, one surgical case, one mental case, and one gynecological case. They are also required to perform one operation on the cadaver.[2]

The medical school, along with the rest of the University of Havana, was closed for three years prior to the Revolution, and reopened early in 1959 with what could only have been a considerably weakened organization, with just 23 of its original 161-member faculty. Some medical school professors left Cuba during the university's three-year closure, while some of those who remained or joined after the Revolution were fired in a wave of political purges.

An official history of the university states that on May 3, 1959, hearings were opened to "purify" the student body and faculty, with a ten-day deadline given for filing denunciations.[3] The following year, officials of the new revolutionary government suspended thirty-seven professors at the medical school "for not recognizing their authority in a public statement."[4] An emergency medical curriculum, presumably with less stringent standards, was introduced and large numbers of nontraditional students from poorer or rural backgrounds were enrolled in order to staff Cuba's expanding public health service as quickly as possible.

In his work on the history of Cuban medicine, Ross Danielson noted that as the best college prep high schools had all been in Havana, many of these new medical students were academically less prepared than their predecessors, though "ideologically superior and conscious of their role as the youth of the Revolution."[5] To some, the new students seemed thuggish, aggressively looking for counter-revolutionary sympathies among students and faculty. The University of Havana hospital, whose name in Spanish had been Our Lady of Mercy, was renamed Comandante Manuel Fajardo, after a physician-turned-guerrilla who had once treated Fidel Castro and who had died in a shootout with anti-Castro rebels in 1960.[6]

Today Cuba has fourteen internationally accredited medical schools, including an institution for foreign students, the Latin American Medical School (ELAM), established in 1999.[7] The curriculum was revised and somewhat abridged and now consists of two years of basic medical science, two years of clinical studies with rotations in different specialities, a fifth year of hospital internship and a final, in-service year working in a community health facility. There is no entrance examination, and applicants are considered on the basis of secondary school transcripts and their record of volunteer work. After completing the hospital internship, and passing a state licensing exam, Cuban medical graduates are required to spend two years working in rural areas assigned by the Health Ministry.

Approximately 30 percent of medical graduates go on to specialist residencies of two to four years' duration following their rural medical service. The surgery residence lasts four years, and produces around seventy newly qualified surgeons each year.[8] There is some question as to how much access Cuban surgeons have to the most recent, less invasive surgical techniques and the specialized equipment needed to perform such procedures. A Swiss orthopedic surgeon gave his Cuban counterparts a class in arthroscopic knee surgery during a visit to the city of Ciego de Avila in 2012, and according to the president of Cuba's Sociedad Cubana de Cirugía Endoscópica, some 30,000 to 40,000 endoscopic examinations are carried out each year.[9] But the Canadian charity MEMO donated surgical instruments for transurethral prostate surgery to a hospital in Villa Clara province, and sent a volunteer urologist to teach his Cuban counterparts the proper surgical techniques to be used with the instruments.[10] The charity's newsletter reported that the hospital had also requested its help "with arthroscopy and laparoscopic abdominal surgery."[11]

Some studies have raised issues about Cuban physicians' understanding of more common ailments. Giardiasis is a parasitic infection found in many parts of the world and is especially prevalent in developing countries where sanitation is poor. A paper published in the *Revista Cubana de Medicina* surveyed sixty-five specialists and twenty-four residents in six different fields in Havana hospitals and polyclinics and reported deficient knowledge of the symptoms and means of infection, with only 36 percent able to adequately define giardiasis and correct answers were given to fewer than half of the questions asked. The researchers concluded that "academic intervention emphasizing formative features related to parasitic diseases in general and giardiasis in particular" was needed.[12]

Cuban doctors do not have much access to international medical journals in print and online, the latter situation a result of the country's limited Internet service. Until 2013 the World Health Organization provided Cuba with the online full-text articles from more than 2,000 foreign medical journals at a modest cost, which otherwise would have been unaffordable, according to Mikhail Benet, chair of the Cuban Medical Journals Advisory Committee. But since then the WHO declared Cuba ineligible for this service, "ironically due to the country's rise in the Human Development Index," he said.[13]

The Castro government has offered free or low-cost medical education to increasing numbers of students from developing countries and more recently, to students from the United States and other Western countries who promise to work in underserved communities after graduation. Cuban medical schools graduated 422 doctors and 67 dentists from developing countries from 1981 to 1985 and by the 1990–1991 academic year this figure had grown to 3,587 foreign doctors and health technicians, mostly from Latin America and sub-Saharan Africa.[14] In 2013, nearly 10,500 students graduated from Cuban medical schools, including 4,843 foreign students from 70 different countries.[15]

Cuba also has bilateral agreements with sympathetic countries to train medical students, with some of the expenses paid for by the students' own governments. In 1995 South Africa signed an agreement to send students to Cuban medical schools, as part of an effort to expand health services in the face of a growing population and increasing number of patients with HIV and related illnesses. South Africa has eight medical schools which graduate around 1,200 new doctors annually and a doctor-to-patient ratio of 57 per 10,000 inhabitants, compared to Cuba's 67.2 doctors per 10,000 inhabitants, and in rural communities the shortage of doctors and other health professionals is especially severe.

According to Africa Health Placements, a nonprofit organization seeking to recruit medical personnel to rural communities, half of those graduating from South African medical schools end up working overseas. Of those South African doctors remaining in the country only a quarter work in public health facilities, mostly in urban areas.[16]

Dr. Godisamang Desmond Kegakilwe, a South African physician who chairs the Rural Doctors Association of Southern Africa, was one of the early participants in this program. He arrived in Sagua la Grande, a coastal city in the central province of Villa Clara, in January of 1998. After studying Spanish he moved to the provincial capital of Santa Clara for medical training, which the Cuban government provided free of charge. He said the South African government paid for his transportation, accommodation, and meals.[17] By 2013 a total of 1,344 South Africans were studying medicine in Cuba and 357 had completed their degrees.

A notice published by the Guateng provincial health authority in Johannesburg invited applications to study medicine in Cuba from students who are eighteen to twenty-five and have fulfilled the minimum academic requirements to begin medical studies in South Africa, including sufficiently high scores in English, mathematics, physical sciences, and life sciences. "The department will fully fund a limited number of successful applicants to study medicine in Cuba," the notice said.[18]

Other South African students are required to pay part of the expenses, depending on their family income levels. The family of Shanice Moodley, a student from KwaZulu-Natal, was required to contribute the equivalent of US$4,900 while the South African government awarded a grant of approximately $3,900 for her meals, accommodation, and pocket money for the first year. In 2013 Moodley and nineteen other students quit the Cuban medical training program within two months and returned to South Africa, complaining of crowded and unsanitary living conditions and poor food.[19]

Graduates of Cuban medical schools who wish to work in South Africa must undergo additional training in order to familiarize themselves with the country's burden of disease, including a very high prevalence

HIV/AIDS and tuberculosis and what is the biggest antiretroviral (ARV) treatment program in the world. According to Dr. Elma de Vries, a former chair of the Rural Doctors Association of Southern Africa, one cannot practice medicine in her country without knowing how to manage very ill patients who may be coinfected with both diseases. This additional training program has been developed specifically for medical students returning from Cuba and generally lasts up to two years. She said that a doctor with a South African medical degree is expected to do much more than a general practitioner in Cuba, which has many more specialists.

"For example, a junior doctor in South Africa, doing a community service year, is expected to handle complicated deliveries and to do caesarean sections and give a general anesthetic. In Cuba this work would be done by obstetricians and anesthetists—of which most smaller hospitals in South Africa have none," she said. De Vries said her Cuban-trained colleagues were very good at understanding primary health care and were willing to work in underserved areas struggling to attract doctors.

"But because of the excellent primary health care system in Cuba, students are not exposed to the complications of diabetes, hypertension and ischemic heart disease that we see in South Africa," she said.[20] There have been some efforts to improve the training of South African students at Cuban medical schools, with mixed results. In 2000 the South African Ministry of Health asked its Cuban counterpart to better develop South African students' knowledge of "various nursing procedures, administration of anesthesia and some surgical techniques, such as hernia repair, appendectomy, surgery for ectopic pregnancy and caesarean sections."[21] A project to develop twelve supplementary courses by Cuban experts from three medical schools was less than successful. Less than half of the South African students completed those additional courses and the majority of professors teaching the courses reported that students were uninterested. The professors cited a lack of appropriate teaching materials and said that many South African students "do not understand Spanish-speakers very well" and preferred to spend time with each other rather than Spanish-speaking students. The students themselves reported insufficient practical activities and a disconnect between course content and the health situation in South Africa. A review of the supplementary courses concluded that this last issue could be the underlying cause of the South African students' discouragement, and that a contributing factor might be "teachers lack of familiarity with the setting in which these future professionals will eventually practice."[22]

There are conflicting accounts of how much the Cuban medical training accord is costing the country but South Africa invests about US$60,000 per student over the six-year Cuban program. Some South African health professionals have argued that it would be less expensive to simply expand medical education within the country, with part of the medical training taking place in rural communities, which might encourage more doctors to work in those areas.

Critics in other African countries have accused government officials of underreporting the cost of sending medical students to Cuba. In 2011 Ghanaian president John Dramani Mahana visited Havana and signed an agreement for 250 students to receive medical training in Cuba. While initial reports suggested this agreement meant the students would receive full scholarships, Ghanaian officials later quoted a cost to the government (presumably for travel expenses) of US$2,240 per student per year. A cabinet memo leaked to a Ghanaian newspaper cited a figure ten times that amount, prompting the country's medical association to call for a public review of the program and ask whether the funds might be better spent on improving medical education and infrastructure within Ghana.[23]

In Namibia a proposal to send 100 students to Cuba, at a cost of US$69,000 each for six years of medical training drew fire when critics pointed out that the cost of medical education in South Africa, China, Russia or Bulgaria was at least 30 percent less.[24]

Cuba's international showcase for medical education is the Escuela Latinoamericana de Medicina (ELAM), or Latin American School of Medicine, which opened its doors in 1999 and trains 10,000 to 12,000 students from mostly Latin American and other developing countries. U.S. students have attended ELAM since 2001, following a visit by the Congressional Black Caucus to Havana and a meeting with Fidel Castro, who offered places at the school for students in their district. The Interreligious Foundation for Community Organization (IFCO), also known as Pastors for Peace, arranged the congressional visit and has actively campaigned for an end to U.S. trade sanctions (referred to as "the blockade") and restrictions on travel to Cuba as well as the release of five Cubans convicted of espionage and serving sentences in U.S. prisons. The group handles U.S. applications to ELAM, interviewing and screening candidates, whose applications are then forwarded to the Cuban Interests Section in Washington. According to the IFCO website, U.S. applicants must meet the following requirements:

- Be between the ages of eighteen and twenty-five at the time of application.
- Must have completed the following college-level, pre-med science courses:
-
    - One year of biology with lab (Biology I and II with labs)
    - One year of chemistry with lab (General Chemistry I and II with labs)
    - One year of organic chemistry with lab (Organic Chemistry I and II with labs)

  - One year of physics with lab (Physics I and II with labs)

- Be physically and mentally fit.
- Come from the humblest and neediest communities in the United States
- Be committed to practice medicine in poor and underserved U.S. communities after graduation.[25]

In Brazil, medical students are recruited from the country's Communist Party, the rural landless rights group Movimento Dos Trabalhadores Sem Terra and the Workers' Party. A notice on the Workers' Party web site invites applications for Cuba's Latin American Medical School, with pre-selection criteria slightly different from those listed for U.S. students:

- A maximum age of twenty-five
- A high school diploma and transcript, with courses in physics, chemistry, and biology
- At least two years of party membership and a recommendation letter from a party leader, approved at a party meeting,
- An HIV test certificate, notarized and signed by a physician,
- For women candidates, a pregnancy test certificate, notarized and signed by a physician,
- A certificate of physical and mental health, notarized and signed by a physician,
- A criminal records check

The Workers' Party international relations department then chooses candidates, whose nominations are later forwarded to the Cuban Embassy. Those chosen are provided with free tuition. Accommodation, food, and travel within Cuba are provided by the Cuban government, but students must arrange their own air travel to and from the country.[26]

Foreign medical students are given placement tests in biology, chemistry, organic chemistry, physics, and Spanish upon their arrival, and some are placed in one or two semester preparatory science programs, along with an intensive Spanish language course lasting twelve weeks. The curriculum is similar to that of other Cuban medical schools and includes practicum placements in a regional polyclinic and a family doctor practice during the first two years. According to the IFCO, the attrition rate of 20 percent at ELAM is similar to dropout rates at other medical schools.[27]

Living conditions for students are spartan, almost as if the experience of poverty is intended as part of their education. All first- and second-year and pre-med students are required to live on the ELAM campus, with no provisions made for married students or those with children. Melissa Mitchell, an American student, shared a crowded room with twenty other students who slept on bunk beds. There was one bathroom containing ten sinks, ten toilets (without seats), and ten showers shared among 120 students, and only cold water which was cut off at night and turned on again in the morning. Students were confined to the school's walled compound during the week, and allowed to leave on weekends only if they had not broken any rules and had successfully completed their course work. There were monthly rations of two toilet paper rolls, two bars of soap, and a pack of sanitary napkins for women, but sometimes even these basic supplies were scarce. The food served to the students was meager+ as well.

"When I first got there, it was rice and beans every day," she told the *Washington Post*. "Then after a while they didn't have beans, and had soup instead, and I'd be like, I'd just die for some beans. I'd be hungry before lunch, and walk out of lunch hungry. But after a while your body gets used to eating less, and you don't want as much." Food was slightly better at the student dormitories at the Salvador Allende hospital, where Mitchell was moved after completing her second year, with chicken served one night a week.[28]

It is unclear whether the actual medical instruction at ELAM is overtly ideological, and some students have maintained there was no pressure to show support for the Castro government. Jamar Williams, a student from Brooklyn, told the *New York Times* that no one is asked to be political. "It's your choice. Many students decide to be political. They go to rallies and read political books. But you can lie low."[29]

An incident reported in a cable from the U.S. Interests Section (USINT) in Havana suggests that foreign medical students in Cuba may in fact find it difficult to maintain a neutral stance. The cable, released by Wikileaks and dated November 11, 2007, states that Pastors for Peace director Reverend Lucius Walker had issued a warning to American medical students during one of his visits to Havana:

> In the past Walker has complimented and encouraged the students but this year Walker spent over an hour warning students against having contact with USINT. He threatened that Pastors for Peace would consider withdrawing scholarships to students who contacted USINT and said that "we would like you to support this government (the Cuban government) but we demand that you at least remain neutral." 2. (C) The student said that he suspects that the change in tone is the result of a letter that he recently wrote to the five Cuban spies currently incarcerated in the United States. The student says that after being repeatedly asked to write an encouraging letter to the five he decided to write a letter in which he attacked the Cuban government for holding political prisoners and asked the five to join him in demanding not only their own freedom, but also the freedom of all political prisoners in Cuba. The student says that within hours many of his classmates, including his American classmates, confronted him with remarks that he made in the supposedly sealed letter. 3. (C) The student said that he felt that his fellow students were generally intimidated by the speech and that he believed that they will avoid contact with the section in the future. He

> said that he doubted that any students would attend a USINT hosted Christmas dinner for the medical students. The student and several classmates attended a Christmas dinner with the Consul General and consular officers last year. 4. (C) The student said that he fears for his own, and his third country national wife's, scholarships. He said that he will continue to serve as a warden and to come to USINT to use the internet and receive newspapers but that he will limit his contact with USINT officials to protect the five years he and his wife have invested in their medical education.[30]

ELAM and thirteen other Cuban medical schools are recognized by the Foundation for Advancement of International Medical Education and Research (FAIMER) and many countries require foreign medical graduates to show a diploma from a FAIMER-listed medical school before taking the licensing examinations necessary to practice medicine. But how well do graduates of Cuban medical schools do on these examinations?

In the United States, where one out of every four doctors was trained overseas, the available data suggests that, on average, Cuban medical school graduates do not perform quite as well on average as other foreign graduates seeking to practice medicine in the country. The Educational Commission on Foreign Medical Graduates (ECFMG) certifies those seeking to take the third step of the three-step United States Medical Licensing Exam, and provided the following figures on graduates of Cuban medical schools applying for certification. Table 5.1 lists the numbers of graduates—Cuban, American and third-country citizens—who graduated from Cuban medical schools and registered for ECFMG certification over a twenty-year period, plus the percentage these Cuban medical school graduates represent out of the total number of foreign medical graduates who registered that year.

Table 5.1. Initial ECFMG Registrants (Cuban Medical School)

Obs	*app_year*	*COUNT*	*PERCENT*
1	1993	91	3.18516
2	1994	137	4.79524
3	1995	212	7.42037
4	1996	260	9.10046
5	1997	243	8.50543
6	1998	181	6.33532
7	1999	92	3.22016
8	2000	88	3.08015
9	2001	94	3.29016
10	2002	135	4.72524
11	2003	133	4.65523

Obs	app_year	COUNT	PERCENT
12	2004	148	5.18026
13	2005	127	4.44522
14	2006	147	5.14526
15	2007	128	4.48022
16	2008	147	5.14526
17	2009	115	4.02520
18	2010	115	4.02520
19	2011	118	4.13021
20	2012	146	5.11026

Table 5.2 shows the number of Cuban medical school graduates who passed the United States Medical Licensing Exam's two-part clinical knowledge examination and a separate clinical skills exam within the required two-year period following their registration with the ECFMG, and the percentage this group represents within the total number of foreign medical graduates certified. They are not necessarily the same applicants who started the process that year.

Table 5.2. ECFMG Certificants (Cuban Medical Schools)

Obs	yearcert	COUNT	PERCENT
1	1993	20	1.6116
2	1994	16	1.2893
3	1995	15	1.2087
4	1996	42	3.3844
5	1997	53	4.2707
6	1998	102	8.2192
7	1999	39	3.1426
8	2000	38	3.0620
9	2001	42	3.3844
10	2002	50	4.0290
11	2003	80	6.4464
12	2004	49	3.9484
13	2005	133	10.7172
14	2006	110	8.8638
15	2007	78	6.2853
16	2008	59	4.7542
17	2009	101	8.1386
18	2010	74	5.9629

Obs	*yearcert*	*COUNT*	*PERCENT*
19	2011	75	6.0435
20	2012	65	5.2377

Comparing the total number of Cuban medical school graduates who register (2,857) with those Cuban medical graduates who pass the exams (1,241) over the twenty-year period listed would suggest a pass rate of 43.4 percent. According to ECFMG spokesman Bill Kelly, slightly more than half of all foreign medical graduates who register pass the qualifying exams.[31]

In Chile, foreign medical school graduates must pass the Examen Unico Nacional de Conocimientos de Medicina (EUNACOM) in order to work in public hospitals, in primary care settings, or to take specialist training. The process includes a written, multiple choice test of 180 questions covering internal medicine, pediatrics, obstetrics and gynecology, surgery, psychiatry, public health, and some specialist topics in opthamology, dermatology, and ear, nose, and throat.[32] EUNACOM figures for Cuban medical graduates taking this part of the examination are as follows:

Table 5.3.

Year	Number of applicants tested from Cuban medical schools	Number of those passing the test
2009	192	89
2010	150	11
2011	164	25

There is also a test of clinical skills covering the areas of medicine, surgery, obstetrics, and pediatrics and according to EUNACOM director Dr. Beltran Mena, the pass rate for all foreign–trained doctors in recent years is 39 percent, and of the 264 Chilean graduates of Cuban medical schools, 28 percent have been approved.[33]

Brazil also requires foreign-trained physicians to take a revalidation exam in order to practice medicine in the country, with an exception made for those participating in the government's Mais Medicos (More Doctors) program to place foreign physicians in underserved areas, which began in 2013. While those doctors educated in Cuba form the second largest group seeking certification, the pass rate for the 2011–2012 period was only 11 percent, according to figures from the Brazilian Ministry of Education. Only a minority of foreign-trained physicians seem to pass the exam, with those educated in Venezuela having the highest pass rate (26 percent), followed by Argentina (22 percent) and Colombia (19 percent).[34] In 2011 Brazil's health minister, Dr. Alexandre Padilha, met with Brazilian students at ELAM to discuss additional medical study at Brazilian universities to improve their chances of passing the licensing exam when they returned home.[35]

NOTES

1. Gaston De Cardenas and Ricardo Puerta, *Cuba, Medicina y Salud: análisis de las condiciones antes y después de la Revolución* (n. p.: Miami, 1993).
2. I. F. Rodriguez Molina, "Medical Education in Cuba," *Southern Medical Journal*, Vol. 23, No. 3 (March 1930).
3. Ramon De Armas, Eduardo Torres-Cuevas, and Ana Cairo Ballester, *Historia de la Universidad de la Habana, Vol. 2, 1930–78* (Havana: Editorial de Ciencias Sociales, 1984), p. 744.
4. Ibid, p.755
5. Ross Danielson, *Cuban Medicine* (New Brunswick, NJ: Transaction Books, 1979), p. 138.
6. De Armas, op. cit., p. 759.
7. The World Health Organization-affiliated AVICENNA directory of medical schools, http://avicenna.ku.dk/database/medicine, lists fourteen Cuban institutions. Other accounts cite as many as twenty-one medical schools plus four higher education medical institutes. The University of Havana was tied for eighty-first place among Latin American universities by the QS world university rankings in 2013.
8. Jose Goderich Latan, "Surgical Education in Cuba," *World Journal of Surgery*, Vol. 34, Issue 5 (May 2010).
9. Luis Hernandez Serrano, "Cuba con mayor cobertura cirugía de mínimo acceso en América Latina," *Juventud Rebelde*, May 21 2010.
10. Interview with MEMO director Dr. Jerome Harvey, June 24, 2013
11. From MEMO's newsletter, November 9, 2011, http://www.memocuba.org/category/trips-to-cuba/
12. Luis Fonte Galindo, Saleh Ali Almannoni, Deisy Martin Pupo, Alexis Monzote Lopez, Lizet Sanchez Valdes, Maria de los Angeles Fernandez, and Irene Fiterre Lancis, "Conocimientos, percepciones y practicas en relación con giardiasis," *Revista Cubana de Medicina*, Vol. 48, No. 4 (October–December 2009).
13. Mikhail Benet, "Cuban Publishing on Primary Health Care: An Inexcusable Absence," *MEDICC Review*, Vol. 15, No. 2 (April 2013).
14. Feinsilver, op. cit., p. 170.
15. Jose A. De la Osa, "Academic Year 2012–2013L 10,500 doctors to gradúate from Cuban universities," *Granma*, June 27, 2013.
16. From Africa Health Placement's web site, http://www.ahp.org.za/donors-and-partners/reports-and-statistics
17. Written correspondence from Dr. Godisamang Desmond Kegakilwe, July 30, 2013. He signed one of his emails with the words, "quiero ser como el che" (I want to be like Che [Guevara]).
18. Guateng province health department bulletin, http://www.health.gpg.gov.za/Pages/STUDYMEDICINEINCUBA(2013).aspx
19. Bongani Hana, "Poor conditions in Cuba bring students home," *Independent Online*, March 25, 2013, http://www.iol.co.za/news/south-africa/kwazulu-natal/poor-conditions-in-cuba-bring-students-home-1.1491242#.UnRPWHCceSo .
20. Written correspondence from Dr. Elma de Vries, July 16, 2013.
21. Frank Quintana, Nelida Sarasa, Oscar Cañizares, Yayly Huguet, "Assessment of a Complementary Curricular Strategy for Training South African Physicians in a Cuban Medical University," *MEDICC Review*, Vol. 14, No. 3 (July 2012), http://www.medicc.org/mediccreview/index.php?issue=21&id=261&a=vahtml.
22. Ibid.

23. Daniel Nonor, "Red Flags over Cuban doctors' scholarship," *The Chronicle* (Accra), May 30, 2012, http://thechronicle.com.gh/red-flags-over-cuban-doctors-scholarship/.
24. Denver Kisting, "Namibia: Cuba Offers Pricey Deal," *The Namibian*, October 2, 2012, http://allafrica.com/stories/201210020497.html?viewall=1.
25. "Frequently Asked Questions," IFCO website, http://www.ifconews.org/node/352. Accessed September 18, 2013.
26. "PT abre pre-selecao para bolsas de Medicina em Cuba," http://www.ptsul.com.br/?doc&mostra&14665. Accessed September 20, 2103.
27. IFCO web site, op. cit.
28. Cindy, Loose, "The Cuban Solution," *Washington Post*, July 23, 2006.
29. *New York Times*, December 8, 2006
30. "Cable: Pastors of Peace warn students against contact with U.S. Interests Section in Cuba," November 30, 2007, published online, http://www.mcclatchydc.com/2011/07/08/117289/cable-pastors-of-peace-warn-students.html.
31. Written correspondence with Bill Kelly of the Educational Commission on Foreign Medical Graduates (ECFMG), September 26, 2013.
32. "Composición de preguntas del EUNACOM-ST," from EUNACOM's website, http://www.eunacom.cl/contenidos/ponderacionesDetalle.pdf.
33. Written correspondence with EUNACOM director Dr. Beltran Mena, November 4, 2013.
34. Jose Alberto Gutiérrez, "Medicos graduados en Cuba, descalificados en pruebas en Brasil," *Café Fuerte*, October 3, 2013, http://cafefuerte.com/cuba/7715-medicos-graduados-en-cuba-descalificados-en-pruebas-en-brasil/.
35. "Acordo facilita revalidação de diplomas médicos obtidos em Cuba," *Saúdenet*, September 26, 2011, http://www.isaude.net/pt-BR/noticia/21175/profissao-saude/acordo-facilita-revalidacao-de-diplomas-medicos-obtidos-em-cuba.

SIX

Research and Pharmaceuticals: "Necessity is the Mother of Invention"

In Habana Vieja, the Cuban capital's partially restored historic center, the Farmacia Taquechel is both a museum and functioning pharmacy. Founded in 1898, it now sells homeopathic products made in Cuba, displayed in glass cabinets underneath long wooden counters. A chandelier hangs from a high ceiling with decorative moldings. The shelves along the walls hold apothecary jars made of French porcelain, which once contained a rich variety of medicines, all made in Cuba. Control and management of the Farmacia Taquechel may be communist, but the atmosphere is Belle Epoch.

Let us step back in time. What would one have seen in Cuba prior to 1958?

One would have seen a pharmaceutical sector with hundreds of pharmaceutical companies, each small and each with its own production facilities and each with its own distribution channels. All of this activity was unregulated.[1] Middle-class and affluent Cubans would have enjoyed access to these products, but the country's poor had to make do with home remedies, if anything.[2] As the government headed by Fidel Castro took hold, Cuban authorities took to nationalizing the hundreds of pharmaceutical companies in Cuba but also began to develop a public national pharmaceutical industry.[3] Cuba also began to train a new generation of scientists and engineers.[4] Today there are approximately 20,000 scientists and an additional 37,500 researchers and technicians working in the biotechnology and pharmaceutical sector.[5]

Cuba went beyond nationalizing these small companies. Fidel Castro began to focus on the pharmaceutical sector as potentially playing a key role in the development of the Cuban economy, earning hard currency while also meeting the domestic needs of its population. In 1972, the government established MediCuba, a government enterprise set up to import and export pharmaceutical and medical equipment. MediCuba worked to reduce the country's reliance on imported pharmaceuticals focusing, rather, on importing base chemicals to be used in pharmaceutical production within Cuba. As a result of these efforts, finished pharmaceutical imports were reduced to the point that they made up only 18 percent of total pharmaceuticals used.[6]

A major turning point in the development of the pharmaceutical industry can be traced to a meeting that occurred in 1980 between Fidel Castro and Dr. Richard Lee Clark, an oncologist and president of the world-renowned MD Anderson Hospital in Houston, Texas, the first American hospital dedicated to the treatment of cancer. Dr. Clark was in Cuba after visiting the laboratories of Dr. Kari Cantell in Helsinki, Finland. Dr. Cantell, internationally known in medical research, was the first scientist able to successfully isolate interferon from human cells.[7] Fidel Castro and Dr. Clark discussed the use of interferon as an approach to fighting cancer and, according to some accounts, it was a result of this meeting that Castro made the strategic decision to develop the biotechnology industry in Cuba.[8] Two of Cuba's top scientists visited MD Anderson Hospital at the invitation of Dr. Clark.[9] Subsequently, in 1981, a team of Cuban scientists led by Manuel Limonta, traveled to Helsinki to Dr. Cantell's laboratory to study how to isolate interferon and produce it in significant quantities. The visit was inspirational to Cuba's scientific and political leadership.[10]

Upon their return to Cuba, the scientific team began to work on converting an old villa into a laboratory; a facility that was to become known as "House #149." The initial concern of this team's scientific efforts was an outbreak of dengue fever in 1981.[11] The development of the pharmaceutical sector was about to begin in earnest. In 1981, the "Biological Front" was established, with the mission of serving as a forum for scientists, engineers, and technicians from a wide range of disciplines to come together for the purpose of further developing the biotechnology industry. What followed was extensive and rapid development of a number of highly active, and soon to be prestigious, biotechnology centers and institutions, organizations that were supposed to work in an integrated, knowledge sharing, noncompetitive structure. The Cuban government believed that there was to be a significant positive outcome resulting from this structure, an outcome that the Cuban government was to proudly emphasize. Whereas, in a market-based economy, firms such as pharmaceutical companies compete with one another, and each firm focuses on those products which best serve its owners and stockholders from a profitability perspective, the Cuban government believed that it could concentrate on those pharmaceutical products that would best meet the needs of the population regardless of profitability. As such, the pharmaceutical industry in Cuba integrated its knowledge-sharing horizontally across pharmaceutical institutes and centers. It also created a vertically integrated structure, a structure which is designed to ensure that research and development activities also integrate with production, provision of information to pharmacists and medical providers, as well as looking beyond the domestic market and its needs in order to enhance global marketing and distribution. The latter activity was structured to earn hard currency as well as to build up relationships with those developing nations perceived to share the Castro government's vision.

The Cuban government invested nearly $1 billion U.S. dollars in the pharmaceutical sector, so that by the 1990s, Cuba found that it could meet 80 percent of its domestic needs, according to the Pan American Health Association.[12] It had succeeded in developing its pharmaceutical exports sector as strategically planned. The value of Cuba's medical product exports increased from $11 million in 1985 to $70 million in 1992.[13] By 1993, Cuba had developed its exports to the point that they generated $100 million annually in revenue, drawing from 1,150 biological and diagnostic products, 132 generic pharmaceuticals and 30 over-the-counter drugs.[14] This figure was to reach $300 million annually by 2005[15] and $405 million in pharmaceuticals and biotechnology products today.[16]

Currently, there are ten major research centers in Cuba, each with its own focus, along with more than fifty research institutions that are associated with these research centers, with approximately 1,500 active scientists working with these institutions.[17]

The premier institution, as well as the first of the major biotechnology centers to be established in Cuba is the Center for Genetic Engineering and Biotechnology (CIGB). The CIGB has 550 active scientists and engineers.[18] As is common with many of these institutions, vertical integration is part of the strategy. The center established a marketing subsidiary, Heber Bintec, in 1991. Heber has successfully marketed products of the center globally, and has established joint ventures with biotechnology companies in China and India. CIGB is perhaps best known for utilizing genetic engineering methodologies to develop the first vaccine which utilized a synthetic antigen to combat Haemophilus Influenza Type B. Interferon is another product produced by the CIGB, influenced in turn, by the earliest scientific interactions associated with the revolution.[19]

In 1991, the Finlay Institute was established, named after one of Cuba's greatest scientists, Dr. Carlos Finlay, who first wrote on the role of biovectors in spreading disease, demonstrated the relationship between mosquitos as carriers, and the outbreak of yellow fever. By understanding the relationship, public health policy could move toward eradicating and preventing yellow fever, as well as controlling other mosquito borne diseases such as malaria and dengue fever (the latter with mixed success). Dr. Finlay's accomplishments have been honored with a prominent statue of the doctor outside the institute. The institute continues to be widely recognized for its research, development and production of vaccines. With a staff of 900 employees, approximately 500 of whom are scientists, the institute has developed and produced more than one-third of the total number of vaccines in Cuba. A reflection of the non-competitive collegial approach that exists among biotech/pharmaceutical companies in Cuba, the Finlay Institute worked collaboratively with other research centers in Cuba in the development of a vaccine that protects against diphtheria, tetanus, pertussis (whooping cough), for both adults and children. A vaccine to prevent hepatitis B (HEBERBIOVAC–HB) has become a major export as well as one that when mixed in combination, becomes a vaccine to prevent all four diseases.[20]

These multiple disease vaccines ease the process and cost of vaccinations in developing countries. Perhaps the most important pharmaceutical development by the Finlay Institute was the world's first effective vaccine against meningitis, VA-MENGOC-BC. It is used against both meningitis B and C. Additional vaccines have been developed by the Finlay Institute including vaccines that fight leptospirosis, typhoid fever, and tetanus.

In 1994, the Center for Molecular Immunology (CIM) was established with a focus on the creation of antibodies for diagnosing and treating cancers.

As with the Finlay Institute, the CIM established a marketing subsidiary, CIMAB.S.A. CIMAB.S.A. has entered into joint ventures globally, including with YM Bioscience, Inc., in Canada, the Center of International Science in China, and Biocom in India. In one of the rare exemptions from the trade restrictions imposed by the United States, the U.S. company, CancerVax, received a license from the U.S. Department of the Treasury in 2003 to work with CIM to undertake clinical trials for a cancer treatment to be used in the United States.[21] This was indeed a reflection of the perceived quality of the biotechnology industry in Cuba, although subsequent clinical trials failed to prove the treatment's efficacy.

The National Center for Bio Products (CNB) is known for its work in bioreagents. The CNB worked together with the CIGB to develop and produce the hepatitis B recombinant vaccine. The CNB has also developed vaccines to simultaneously inoculate against numerous disease processes. A vaccine to deal with allergies and a product developed to treat anemia also came out of the facilities of the CNB. CNB, with its six research and production facilities, is able to produce 14,000 doses of vaccines per hour. The products of CNB are used domestically and exported globally.[22]

One institution which predates the revolution and is still operating today is the Pedro Kouri Tropical Medicine Institute (IPK). The IPK dates back to 1937 and is a part of the University of Havana School of Medicine.[23] Pedro Kouri Esmeja, the founder of the institute and a professor of parisitology and diseases, focused his work on parasites, and was the founder of the *Journal of Laboratory and Clinical Parasitology* in 1935. The

IPK has worked on serious medical issues in the region including dengue fever and tropical parasites. More recently, this teaching facility has also turned its attention to infectious diseases such as HIV.[24]

A number of centers work on diagnostic and medical services and equipment. The Center for Immunology (CIE) develops testing kits for infectious diseases and has a marketing division which markets and distributes globally. The National Center for Neurosciences focuses on medical equipment for neurological issues.[25]

The National Center for Scientific Research (CNIG) is a research laboratory established in 1965 which develops medical diagnostic equipment as well as pharmaceuticals.[26] One of its products and major exports, PPG-5, is an auto-diabetic and cholesterol-lowering drug made from sugarcane, plentiful in Cuba. Its launch was marked by controversy, as some of the drug's promoters also claimed it had aphrodisiac effects and should be marketed as such.

Dr. Hilda Molina, one of the founders of Cuba's Centro Internacional de Restauración Neurológica (CIREN), said she and her colleagues held monthly meetings with researchers from the biotech center, which were often attended by Fidel Castro himself. According to Molina, the drug's cholesterol-lowering properties had been clinically proven, but not its claim to enhancing sexual potency. Nevertheless, Castro considered it "a veritable gold mine" and wanted to introduce PPG-5 to the world market as soon as possible, selling it in all the country's airports (presumably without a prescription): "We have to develop an intense campaign aimed at tourists knowing the effects of PPG on cholesterol and sexual potency, We have to ask the foreign entrepreneurs who have invested here to introduce PPG in their countries," she quotes him as saying. "And all the companeros who travel abroad, whatever their mission is, should take PPG and get their counterparts to not only get interested in this medication, but to help us distribute it and propagandize its benefits."[27]

Other research scientists who defected after working in Cuba's biotech industry said that many of the clinical trials undertaken were enough to prove some effect, but not enough to substantiate later marketing claims or meet the standards of many countries. Dr. Cesar Reynel, who worked at the sector in the early 1990s, said there was a tendency to inflate results, following "a very old rule in Cuba that if the results are favorable, increase them by one zero." "There is no independent government body to oversee this research, and no safe way for a whistleblower to report wrongdoing," he said.[28]

Dr. Jose de la Fuente, former director of research at the CIBG, said that in the beginning the establishment of an advanced scientific center in Havana had been the most rewarding endeavor he and other young Cuban scientists had ever undertaken, but the sector later experienced increasing institutional and political paralysis. The industry was overseen by the Secretary of Cuba's State Council, Jose M. Miyar Barrueco, aka

"Chomi," who at Castro's behest insisted on making every administrative and policy decision, even though he had no scientific background. The economic crisis from the loss of Soviet subsidies caused the government to lessen its commitment to scientific research and shift its attention toward tourism. Reduced funding resulted in damaged relationships among the different research centers, with "increasingly fierce competition between groups for resources and paternity rights over promising projects."[29]

According to De la Fuente, the Cuban biotech sector did have some internationally recognized achievements, such as previously mentioned vaccine against hepatitis B and immunological control of tick infestations.[30] The sector also has a number of centers on animal health, including the National Center for the Protection of Laboratory Animals, (CENPALAS), established in 1982, and the National Center for Agricultural and Animal Health (CENSA), established in 1969. For most developing countries, it does not make economic sense for a country to develop and produce its own pharmaceuticals, a reflection of the lack of appropriate economies of scale. Costs are potentially higher and quality lower.[31] It is argued that this is especially true post-2001 when the World Trade Organization passed the Doha Declaration on Public Health which states in part, "WTO members' right to protect public health and, in particular, to promote access to medicine for all," and provides for compulsory licensing of pharmaceuticals in order to protect public health.[32] Yet Cuba produces 80 percent of its pharmaceutical products domestically, importing 40 percent of needed raw materials from China.[33] Cuba is recognized as one of those rare countries where it makes more sense to produce its own drugs rather than import, a result of the lack of hard currency, U.S. trade sanctions, the need to bring in raw materials through expensive air transport, and its ability to produce high quality, highly effective pharmaceuticals at reasonable costs.[34]

Cuba's pharmaceutical sector has developed significant relationships with other countries, which became especially important during and after the Special Period. Joint ventures with other countries have enabled Cuba to access foreign capital, thereby allowing for further development of the pharmaceutical sector. Cuba has developed licensing agreements with firms in Europe to conduct Stage III clinical trials as well.[35] The country has adopted the WTO's Trade-Related Aspects of Intellectual Property Rights (TRIPS)[36] as well as the WTO's vaccine pre-qualifications requirements. Cuba complies with the International Standardization Organization's (ISO) standards including Good Laboratory Practice (GLP), Good Manufacturing Practice (GMP), and Good Clinical Practice standards (GCP).[37] The pharmaceutical sector in Cuba has developed relationships with firms in countries in Europe, as well as Canada, Mexico, Brazil, China, and India.[38] Export markets have included Argentina, Colombia, Mexico, Russia, and a number of countries in Asia. Cuba has had a history of undertaking trade, barter, and marketing relationships with other countries. For example, Cuba established a trade relationship with the Ukraine. Common pharmaceuticals were traded for agriculture commodities. With Iran, the trade agreement has involved pharmaceutical products (together with medical professionals and sugar) for oil.[39] To celebrate Cuba's twenty-fifth anniversary recognizing the People's Republic of China in 1959, Cuba and China established the joint Chinese-Cuban Biotech Pharmaceutical Company, the doors were opened in September 2005. One of the products that was developed and produced was TheraCIM h-R3 to treat neck and head cancer.[40]

Not all of the joint ventures that Cuba entered into were successful. For example, a joint venture that Cuba with Brazil's Fundación Oswaldo Cruz (FIOCRUZ), to manufacture and distribute antimeningitis pharmaceuticals, did not have this level of success. A dispute occurred between the two countries relating to the price and the perceived quality of the vaccine. Brazil ultimately agreed to purchase the vaccine directly from Cuba on an as need basis at those times when a meningitis outbreak actually occurred.[41]

A most recent development regarding the support for pharmaceuticals and biotechnology advances involves an integrated and market focused approach to research, development, production, and marketing. The Ministry of Economy and Planning (MEP) has worked to form BioCubaFarma. BioCubaFarma is the result of a merger of the pharmaceutical sector, under the umbrella of the Corporación Quimefa with its approximately sixty pharmaceutical research, development, production, and marketing groups and its biotechnology counterpart sector under the direction of the Polo Científico del Oeste, again, responsible for research, development, production, and marketing.

The merged entity includes thirty-eight research and development centers, sixteen production entities, nineteen firms responsible for marketing and three service providers. According to Cuban officials, BioCubaFarma provides for 90 percent of the pharmaceutical needs of Cuba.[42]

BioCubaFarma's stated mission is to develop and produce medicines, equipment, and high technology devices to improve the health of the people, utilize advances in food production, and provide goods and services for export.[43] BioCubaFarma has been developed to work as a business entity. It is not managed or subsidized by the Cuban government. The intent is to generate profits for biotechnology and pharmaceuticals. The concept is to focus on business methodologies of process improvement and improved performance outcomes, including monitoring and managing of quality indicators and production capacity. There is to be a strategic plan with the goal of putting into place policies to spur research and development of medicines and high tech products and services, as well as, negotiation and enforcement of foreign trade and technology transfer. Intellectual direction is to be provided by the Centro de Estudios

Avanzados de Cuba (Center for Advanced Studies of Cuba, CEAC). The organizational structure is to be guided by a Senior Business Management Organization with the chairperson of the organization chosen by the Council of Ministers.[44]

Much of health care in Cuba is paternalistic in nature. Patients may be injected with medications without knowing what is in the syringe, thereby overriding the patient's individual decision making process. Such activities often have a political motive. Decisions made regarding anything from sterilization of the mentally ill to the "therapeutic" abortion of medically compromised fetuses is done to assure that the statistical outcomes regarding the health status of the country look good.[45] Thus the question arises as to whether a culture exists for the violation of individual rights when it comes to medical research and clinical trials associated with the significant pharmaceutical industry sector in Cuba. At the same time, the Cuban government has a strong interest in marketing its products overseas, and clinical trials are sometimes undertaken overseas involving joint ventures. For example, the cancer drug, Nimotuzumab, used for advanced stage cancer of the head, neck, and brain, was developed in Cuba's Center of Molecular Immunology with clinical trials in Europe and Japan, where it can be anticipated that human subjects are afforded appropriate protection.[46]

RETAIL PHARMACIES AND THE ROLE OF THE PHARMACIST

In 1994, Cuba implemented its National Drug Program. The intent was to have pharmaceutical utilization and distribution be part of an integrated health care system. The system of incorporation of pharmaceuticals in the system is tiered, like the health care system in general.

A pharmatherapeutic committee resides at the local level. The role of the committee is both prescriptive and epidemiological. Prescriptions are to be based on the evaluation and assessment of a patient and his/her record by a specialist. Nearly all pharmaceutical drugs require a prescription. Prescribed medications are subsequently dispersed through a local area pharmacy to which each individual is assigned. The committee also reviews the long-term pharmaceutical use by chronically ill patients.[47]

The pharmatherapeutic committee works with the "Essential Drug List" as recommended by the World Health Organization. The Ministry of Health (MINSAP) established a basic list of pharmaceutical drugs (BDL) in 1991, a list which has shortened over time. Thus, in 1996, there were 916 pharmaceutical drugs on the BDL. Of these, 290 were considered in short supply and 73 were incorporated into the card control system. Four years later, the number of pharmaceutical drugs on the BDL had decreased to 804, of which 200 were in short supply and 59 remained in the card control system.[48] Today there are about 350 pharmaceuticals on the BDL.

Within the Ministry of Health, the Center for the Development of Pharmacoepidemiology (CDP) utilizes the National Pharmacoepidemiology Network. The network has multiple objectives. At the national policy level, the network is the vehicle by which the government interacts with, and regulates the domestic pharmaceutical manufacturing and marketing sector. The network has also been responsible for monitoring domestic pharmaceutical utilization, effectively and proactively disseminating information, and providing ongoing training to the pharmacist and medical professional community.[49] The network developed a therapeutic guide for physicians in 1995. Since 1998, the network has provided an annual update on treatments as well as a significant number of teleconferences relating to appropriate and new pharmaceutical regimens. Scientific meetings are held regularly for the pharmacoepidemiological profession. Research discussed at these conferences includes focus on the effects of different drug regimens for different disease processes, adverse drug events and adverse drug interactions, and inappropriate drug use and potential overuse by the elderly.[50] With the very large geriatric population in Cuba, one that is growing significantly over time, traditional and herbal medicine, so-called "green" medicine, has become very important in the prevention and treatment of numerous ailments. Geriatric medicine generally calls for no more than four pharmaceuticals for the elderly. Each pharmaceutical is to be prioritized as to the severity of the medical issue being addressed. It is the interaction of pharmaceutical drugs and the resultant effects on the elderly patient which are often times harmful and potentially deadly.

Pharmaceutical consultation services are available. The CDP has developed and disseminated practice guidelines for the pharmaceutical treatment of a number of chronic disease processes, including hypertension, respiratory disease and distress, and acute and chronic pain. Given that cardiovascular disease is the leading cause of death in Cuba, the CDP has focused much public education and professional training on pharmaceutical maintenance of hypertension, angina, and heart failure. Classes through a continuing education program on pharmaceutical treatment of chronic ailments are offered by the CDP, a program that has been taken by a significant number of physicians over time.[51]

The history of pharmacist training in Cuba is a long one, dating back to 1842, when the University of Havana first formed the Academy of Pharmacy Studies. Official training began in 1863 as a new curriculum was developed. In 1908, an American working in Cuba worked to create the official study, "Pharmacy Practices."[52]

Cuba's Ministry of Health, MINSAP, has taken an active role in assuring an appropriate integrated role for pharmacists.[53] The pharmacist, as part of the local medical team, is involved in assuring that pharmaceutical prescriptions are appropriate and reflect current treatment guidelines. Drug interactions are monitored and adverse reactions to drugs are gauged. These drug interactions include those of herbal and non-traditional derivation as well. The pharmacist also works with the medical team to determine and treat drug addiction, adjust diet, and prescribe modifications in lifestyle, ultimately working to provide effective self-care by the patient/resident.[54] As such, the role of the pharmacist extends far beyond the role in most other countries where the pharmacist is to merely follow the pharmaceutical prescription orders of the physician.

The pharmacist also runs the local pharmacy dispensary, to which each resident in Cuba is assigned to. If a trained pharmacist is not available, an experienced pharmacy technician may run the pharmacy. This extensive, expansive role of the pharmacist requires a significant level of education and training. Pharmacists in Cuba today are trained in pharmacology, pharmaceutical therapy, and delivery systems. Given that pharmacists are responsible for monitoring and managing the medical professional team in herbal medicines and monitoring of all drug interactions, both Western and traditional pharmaceutical medicines are also part of the curriculum. Pharmacist education now also includes analytical and problem solving skills, communication and team-building skills, critical thinking and ethics, and ultimately, leadership training. It is a position that requires monitoring and oversight of population health as well. The position is meant to allow for an understanding of, and commitment to social responsibility.[55] This is all a function of the significant role that the pharmacist specialist plays in the integrated medical team.[56]

Whereas the pharmacist's role in drug dispensing as part of the integrative team is critical, the ability of the pharmacist and, for that matter, the entire health care team, to dispense pharmaceuticals in a safe manner is potentially compromised. A number of eyewitness accounts of conditions associated with injectable pharmaceuticals speak to the lack of available hypodermic needles, syringes, or the sterilization tools and materials necessary to sterilize previously used supplies. Stories speak of sterilization equipment broken, not available, or needles "sterilized" in water as they were being readied for additional use.[57] Use of syringes without appropriate sterilization has been an underlying cause of infectious diseases among the population. This includes syringes used by physicians and nurses as well as local lay practitioners who provide basic health care but who lack training or knowledge of sterilization techniques.[58]

One of the most significant results of the lack of sterilization equipment or techniques was a significant number of cases of cirrhosis of the liver in the 1980s and 1990s. It was determined that these cases were non-A and non-B hepatitis. Once hepatitis C was discovered in the 1990s, it was realized that, indeed, hepatitis C was the underlying disease process. Initially it was baffling to medical providers as those individuals with cirrhosis and hepatitis C were not patients who displayed any of the commonly known risk factors.[59] Additionally, many women now diagnosed with this illness were in their fifties to their seventies and who had emigrated to Miami. These women also exhibited none of the risk factors normally attributed to those with this disease process.[60]

GREEN MEDICINE, BY CHOICE AND NECESSITY

Much has been discussed relating to the public use and training of specialist medical providers in herbal and traditional medicine. In 1992, the federal government in Cuba established a policy requiring the integration of natural and traditional medicine with Western pharmaceutical practice.[61] This was a reflection of the pressures put on the Cuban economy and the health care system, by the effects of the Special Period. With the collapse of the Soviet Union, hard currency became in short supply. This aggravated the problem further. As Cuba had difficulty purchasing the pharmaceuticals it needed to meet the needs of its population, it also had difficulty purchasing the raw materials needed to produce the Western medicines that its pharmaceutical industry was capable of producing. In 1995, the Ministry of Health established a commission to evaluate and develop natural and traditional medicine. The tenets of natural and traditional medicine are now taught in every medical school in the country. Components of natural and traditional medicine are utilized in hospitals throughout Cuba. The vast majority of physicians in Cuba incorporate these methods in their practices.[62]

In addition to the underlying political-economic push for integration of herbal and traditional medicine into the treatment regimen in Cuba, there is, independently, a rich history of the use of natural and traditional medicine, so-called green medicine, in Cuba.

Immigrant populations who emigrated to Cuba from countries in Africa (primarily forced emigration from West Africa as slaves), as well as those who emigrated from China, Haiti, India, and Spain, each brought with them a culture, tradition, and knowledge of the use of medicinal plants and herbs.[63] The development of a culture of folk medicine took hold.[64]

The Taíno and Caribe Indians who originally resided on the island prior to European emigration, also influenced the continued use of herbal and plant medicines.[65] The Haitian population that emigrated to Cuba has long used medicinal plants, which have now become part of a Cuban medicinal plant methodology.[66] The Chinese (initially indentured workers who were brought over to work on the plantations in Cuba) brought their practice of traditional Chinese medicine. There have been more modern influences of Chinese medicine as well, such as the medicine of the barefoot doctors of the Communist countries of China, North Korea, and Vietnam that have been introduced to Cuba.[67] The practitioners of traditional, herbal, and plant medicine in Cuba today include the Yerberos, the Curanderos, the root doctors originally from countries in Africa, and the Santerios. As such, there is this strong linkage to folk medicine. Today, Yerberos and Santerios are required to complete a two week course to be licensed by the Cuban Ministry of Health and, as such, are accepted as an integral participant in the provision of health care in the island nation.[68]

The WHO has indicated that traditional medicine includes beliefs, knowledge, and the application through health care that utilizes plant, animal, and mineral therapies. These medicines are used in conjunction with holistic, spiritual, and hands-on methodologies to prevent illness and bring about wholeness, as well as to diagnose and treat as needed.[69]

Herbal and plant medicine is fully integrated into the education, training, and provision of care in the health care system of Cuba. The PAHO has been extremely complimentary of this activity. The integrated medicine approach has allowed for financially reasonable and clinically effective approaches for medicinal use to deal with disease processes affecting the populations of many developing countries.[70] Nevertheless, the director of the WHO, Dr. Margaret Chan, while praising the role and importance of traditional medicine, also provides a word of caution, saying, "traditional medicine has much to offer, but cannot always supply the access to modern drugs and measures that very effectively make the difference between life and death in many millions of people."[71]

General education, medical education, and clinical training oriented toward the prescribing and use of natural or green medicine, and its integration with traditional medicine, begins already in the K–12 school system.[72] The typical medical student, already exposed to the basics, now receives significant exposure to the field of natural medicine during his/her typical six-year program. By the early part of the twenty-first century, every one of the twenty-three medical schools in Cuba incorporated green medicine in their curriculum. In turn, 86 percent of practicing physicians utilize natural medicine in their provision of service.[73]

Medical students are given exposure to the basics of medicinal plants. In their pharmacology courses, students learn about forty-nine herbal treatments approved by the Cuban Medical Authority. The fourth year of medical school includes additional exposure to herbal medicine. In the fifth and sixth year of medical school, there is in-depth training of Chinese medicine, herbs, and the underlying philosophy of the use of these modalities. The final two years of medical school also include a forty-hour rotation under the direction of natural, traditional medicine specialists.[74]

Upon graduation, there is a two-year medical residency opportunity in the field of "medicina general integral." This residency program, in addition to exploring in-depth alternative medicine, places a strong focus on medicinal plants, their ingredients, biochemical impacts, and the indications and contraindications of herbal plant medication.[75]

Continuing education associated with specific aspects of natural and traditional medicine is also applied. Those who hold a degree in medicine, nursing, pharmacy, or physical therapy, may also apply for a two-year master's degree that is oriented toward research in natural medicine.[76]

Traditional medicines are well integrated into the treatment protocol. The Essential Drug List, which Cuba has adopted at the suggestion of the WHO, a suggestion made to all countries, contains both Western pharmaceuticals, as well as green medicine.[77] As is true with all Western pharmaceuticals, traditional and natural medicines are supposed to meet international quality standards.[78]

Research, development, and distribution of natural and traditional medicines are an organized part of the pharmaceutical structure in Cuba. Green medicine is incorporated at all levels of Cuba's integrated health care system, from the community family physician through the highest level of tertiary care within hospital facilities. The Ministry of Health has set minimum standards.[79]

At the community level, family physicians and nurses utilize natural medicine as part of their practice. Physicians must have passed a course and are updated regarding green medicine formularies. Nurses who are part of the practice team receive training as well. The medical team provides a feedback loop, utilizing natural medicines in its practice, and in turn, providing information regarding the level of utilization and its relative effectiveness.[80]

Polyclinics, the next level in the provision of care in the country, also include natural medicine, including homeopathic and flower essence treatment as part and parcel of a practice of integrated Western medicine and traditional herbal medicine. As with primary care community providers, physicians and nurses must have successfully completed the basic courses in traditional medicine.[81]

Hospitals in Cuba oftentimes have a "Center for Integrated Development of Natural and Traditional Medicine." Staff is again required to have graduated from the basic courses. An integrative medicine approach is used in conjunction with the center and is required to have a physician who holds a master's degree in traditional and natural medicine. Natural pharmaceuticals are prescribed in conjunction with natural medical services which may include tai chi, yoga, surgical acupuncture, magnets, suction cups, and other aspects of traditional and oriental medicine techniques.

In the tertiary hospital system, Cuba incorporates the provincial Centers for the Development of Natural and Traditional Medicine. So, as is true with other aspects of medical and health care, the exploration and provision of traditional medicine and pharmaceuticals is reflective of the tiered and integrated approach. At this higher level of care, traditional and herbal medicine and oriental medicine techniques are integrated with Western medicine and pharmaceutical treatment. These facilities, in addition, have laboratories to produce and evaluate.[82]

The scientific evaluation of herbal medicine, including cost effectiveness, contraindications, and dosing, is overseen by the Cuban government.[83] Within the Ministry of Public Health of Cuba, the Municipal Home Pharmacy Network (MHPN) oversees the use of drugs in each territory, including drugs produced outside Cuba and natural and traditional medicines. The Center for the Development of Pharmacoepidemiology (CDA), coordinates activities of the provincial networks of pharmacoepidemiology. The CDA reports to the First Deputy Minister of the Public.[84]

With the rich and extensive multiethnic roots of traditional, herbal, and folk medicine in Cuba, the development of a complex mix of traditional medicine is not surprising. At last count, there were nearly 200 herbal and traditional medicine formulations utilizing nearly as many plants.[85]

Traditional medicines utilize plants and herbs, but also incorporate other elements, including animal byproducts and manufactured ingredients. The list of possible ingredients is extensive, and the Cuban government has taken on active development and assessment of these formulas, doing common pharmacological studies, but also phytochemical and ethnobotanical studies.[86]

The variety of ingredients in these formulations is quite interesting and, most probably, not all of these ingredients have been incorporated in the studies and evaluations by the Cuban government. In an assessment of ingredients used in medicinal formulations used typically in the eastern part of Cuba, Cano and Volpato found the following variety of ingredients used in these herbal medicines:

> Aspirins, beer, bee's honey, bovine lung, castor oil, condensed milk, cricket's legs, dried cod liver oil, dry wine (not necessarily grape wine), duck's eggs, Epsom salts, fat of majá, goat's excrement, goat's hoof, magnesium powder, mule's hoof, nest of comején (American termite), rum, salt (sodium chloride), sugar, sweet wine (not necessarily of grapes), tincture of iodine, tobacco's tops, urine of the mother of the person being sick, vinegar, whale's sperm, wheat meal, yolk of hen's eggs."[87]

Many of these formulations are used nationally and are part of the basic herbal and traditional medicine methodologies known throughout the country. These formulations will tend to use plants and herbs cultivated in Cuba but may be combined with plants and herbs imported from Asia and Europe. Other formulations are unique to and known only in a limited area of Cuba and the plants used in the process are wild in the area.[88]

The majority of formulations are associated with specific disease processes or symptoms. Thus the stomach and digestive system have nineteen folk and herbal medicinal treatments. The liver and related issues are treated with fourteen folk and herbal medicines. Kidney problems are treated with sixteen folk and herbal medicines and rheumatoid conditions are treated with ten of these formulations. Respiratory ailments are treated with thirty-eight and diabetes by nine. Similarly, skin issues are treated with ten formulations; nervousness and insomnia with nine; parasites, fifteen; gynecological issues, ten; fever (including malaria), five; and the broad category of other afflictions by twenty-two.[89]

The majority of these formulas use a combination of two to three plants. Approximately a quarter use four to five plants, the remaining formulas using six or more plants (one formula uses nineteen plants), and many of these plant formulas are dosed as per experience and custom.[90] The large majority of these are processed as liquid preparations. Others are mixed with oils as topical treatments or as aromatherapy. All parts of the plants are ultimately used.[91]

Many of the herbal and plant preparations are formulated in the home environment. Those that are complicated to prepare are generally those that require the certified Yerbero. There has been a lot of focus on Cuba regarding "therapeutic" abortion to reduce the risk of infant mortality or compromised births. Obstetricians are more focused on using Western methods, but there is a long tradition of using herbs to induce abortion in Cuba. These methods predate even the arrival of Europeans, and were used by Taino and Caribe Indians.[92] In contrast, to counter impotence or sterility, a combination of plants and food items such as eggs, milk, and wine, are used as a remedy.[93] There are fermented drinks with certain African ethnic roots that are bottled with numerous herbal and plant components, called galones.[94] These preparations use a tiered approach. The base level of the galón uses three ingredients considered to be magic plants: roots of Cocos nucifera, Erythroxylum havanense, and Roystonea regia as a stimulant and to counter bacteria.[95]

The Afro-Cuban background adds a second level of ingredients that allows the preparation to be directed toward specific disease processes.[96] Several of these species are used globally for a variety of venereal diseases including the treatment of acute syphilis.[97]

There are a number of plants that are added as a third level of specificity, used to generally treat just one disease or used uniquely by a given healer. Roots used medicinally have a strong African medicine base. As a result of the spread of slavery and immigration trends, root medicine became an important form of green medicine. Those who are practitioners of root medicine, usually those of the Afro-American culture, are called "root doctors."[98] Special attention is given to assure that in using the roots, the entire plant is not destroyed.[99]

It is recognized that some of the formulas used have toxins in them. The clay from termite mounds is used as a binder with the toxins in order to remove their toxic effect.[100]

Miel de Güira is perceived to have more of a Caribbean heritage, perhaps associated with pre-European native populations.[101] These are complex mixtures, which tend to use fruit of the güira tree and are mixed with a sweetener such as sugar, honey, or rum. It is considered to have healing properties as a result of its natural chemical compounds. Different mixtures are utilized for different illnesses, symptoms, or health issues. Again, as with previous herbal and plant formulas, one of the areas of focus is sexual health. Depending upon the formulation, it is used to treat gonorrhea (and is commonly used in Haiti and the Dominican Republic for this purpose as well).[102] Given the specific Miel de Güira mixture used, it is intended to regulate the menstrual cycle and can be used for either fostering pregnancy or alternatively, and by contrast, abortion.

Thus, in terms of instructions used with the Miel de Güira formula, it is indicated that one "should then not smell the preparation in order not to loose [sic] the baby."[103] Finally, a type of soy drink, Pru is perceived to have medicinal value as well. It is thought to be of African-Haitian background.[104] It is plant based, fermented and mixed with sugar and is thought to reduce blood pressure.[105]

In 2000, the WHO stated, "The use of herbal medicine is well-established and widely acknowledged to be safe and effective and may be accepted by national authorities."[106] Whereas side effects may be fewer with Western pharmaceuticals, this is not to say that utilizing herbal medicine is without risk. Warnings such as those indicated above as well as deviations from nationally recognized and regulated norms should cause one pause. There is indication of underreporting of adverse effects.[107] Risks associated with natural medicine include use of herbs that are perceived as new to Cuban herbal medicine, and may be drawn from wild as opposed to cultivated sources. Herbal treatments may be used at the local level with no controls for the amount of plant materials used, or the level of toxicity of these ingredients, either in the soils where the plant is drawn from, or in the plant itself.[108] Potency and toxicity may even vary depending upon what time of year the plant is harvested.[109] Further, substitute plant-based medicines are oftentimes used when a given ingredient is in short supply, with the potential for significantly different effects.[110]

Additional risks include drug interactions with both traditional medicine and Western medicine. Finally, the condition of the patient him/herself may impact on the toxicity of an herbal medicine for that person. The elderly as well as those who have chronic illnesses or compromised immune systems may find that cardio, liver, and/or kidney function is adversely affected by herbal medicine.[111] Pregnant women and lactating women and their infants and unborn children are at greater risk.[112] As noted, even the category, Miel de Güira, can either enhance the chances for pregnancy or do the exact opposite, induce abortion, with abortion perceived by herbalists to be possible even from smelling the herbal medication.[113]

NOTES

1. Faraz Vahid Shahidi, "Globalization From Below: Health, Pharmaceuticals, Cuba and Red Scares," *Undercurrent: The Canadian Undergraduate Journal of Development Studies* Vol. 7, No. 2 (2010), pp. 33–39.
2. Robert S. Tancer, "The Pharmaceutical Industry in Cuba," *Clinical Therapeutics* Vol. 17, No. 4 (1995), pp. 791–798.
3. Ibid.
4. Debra Evenson, "Cuba's Biotechnology Revolution," *MEDICC Review* Vol. 9, No. 1 (2007), pp. 8–10.
5. Domingo Amuchastegui, "Cuba seeks to decentralize biotech, pharmaceutical sector," *Cuba News*, February 1, 2013.
6. Tancer, op. cit.
7. Marguerite R. Jiménez, "Cuba's pharmaceutical advantage," *NACLA Report on the Americas* Vol. 44, No. 4 (2011), pp. 26.
8. Ibid.
9. Ibid.
10. Ibid.
11. Simon M. Reid-Henry, *The Cuban Cure: Reason and Resistance in Global Science* (Chicago: University of Chicago Press, 2010).
12. Pan American Health Organization, "Health in the Americas: 2012 Edition," *Regional Outlook and Country Profiles* (Washington, D.C: PAHO, 2012).
13. Tancer, op. cit.
14. Tancer, op. cit.; Evenson, op. cit.
15. Evenson, op. cit.
16. "Cuba increased exports by 20% in 2011 compared to 2010,"*Cubaencuentro*, April 17, 2012.
17. Evenson, op. cit.
18. Ibid.
19. Ibid.
20. Ibid.
21. Ibid.
22. Ibid.
23. Ibid.
24. Ibid.
25. Ibid.
26. Tancer, op. cit.; Evenson, op. cit.
27. Hilda Molina, *Mi Verdad*, (Buenos Aires: Editorial Planeta, 2010), p. 237.
28. Interview with Dr. Cesar Reynel, October 16, 2013.
29. Jose De la Fuente, "Wine into Vinegar—the fall of Cuba's biotechnology," *Nature*, October 2001 and author's interview, November 12, 2013.
30. Ibid.
31. Warren Kaplan and Richard Laing, "Local Production of Pharmaceuticals: Industrial Policy and Access to Medicines. An Overview of Key Concepts, Issues and Opportunities for Future Research," *The World Bank*, (2005), pp. 1–40; Sara Bennett, Jonathan D. Quick, and Germán Velásquez, "Public-Private Roles in the Pharmaceutical Sector-Implications for Equitable Access and Rational Drug Use," *Health Economics and Drug*, EDM Series No. 5 (Geneva: World Health Organization Task Force on Health Economics, 1997).

32. Kaplan and Laing, op. cit.
33. Tancer, op. cit.
34. Kaplan and Laing, op. cit.
35. Jen Plahte and Simon Reid-Henry, "Immunity to TRIPS Vaccine Production and the Biotechnology Incidents in Cuba," in *The New Political Economy of Pharmaceuticals: Production, Innovation, and TRIPS in the Global South*, ed. Hans Lötgren and Owain David Williams. (Basingstoke: Palgrave MacMillan, 2013).
36. "Fact Sheet: TRIPS and Pharmaceutical Patents: Developing countries' transition periods," last modified September, 2006, http://www.wto.org/english/tratop_e/trips_e/factsheet_pharm04_e.htm.
37. Plahte and Reid-Henry, op. cit.
38. Tancer, op. cit.; Evenson, op. cit,
39. Tancer, op. cit.
40. Stephen Millies, "China, Cuba unite to fight disease," *Worker's World*, October 4, 2005.
41. Tancer, op. cit.
42. Amuchastegui, op. cit.
43. "Create a new business group for biotechnology and pharmaceutical activity in Cuba," *Granma*, December 10, 2013.
44. Ibid.
45. Elizabeth Kath, *Social Relations and the Cuban Health Miracle* (New Brunswick, NJ: Transaction Publishers, 2010), pp. 73–129.
46. "Cuba-Investing in Biotechnology to Battle Cancer" *Medical News Today*, February 4, 2013
47. Alina Martínez Sánchez and J. Warren Salmon, "Overview of Complementary/Alternative Medicine in the Cuban Health System," *The International Journal of Healing and Caring*, (2013), pp. 1–20.
48. Eduard Diogène et al., "The Cuban experience in focusing pharmaceuticals policy to health population needs: initial results of the National Pharmacoepidemiology Network (1996–2001)," *Pharmacoepidemiology and Drug Safety* Vol. 12, (2003), pp. 405–7.
49. Ibid.
50. Ibid.
51. Diogène et al., op. cit.
52. Caridad Sedeño Argilagos, "Los prácticos de Farmacia en Cuba desde 1912," *Revista Cubana de Farmacia* Vol. 43, No. 3 (2009).
53. Ministry of Public Health of Cuba, National Medical Records and Health Statistics Bureau, "Annual Health Statistics Report 2005," Havana, Cuba, 2005.
54. Martínez Sánchez and Salmon, op. cit.
55. Ibid.
56. Ibid.
57. Katherine Hirschfeld, *Health, Politics, and Revolution in Cuba since 1898* (New Brunswick, NJ: Transaction Publishers, 2008); Linda M. Whiteford and Laurence G. Branch, *Primary Health Care in Cuba: The Other Revolution* (Lanham: Rowman & Littlefield Publishing Group, 2009).
58. Miguel A. Faria, "Socialized (Free) Medical Care in Cuba (Part I): A Poor State of Health," *Surgical Neurology* Vol. 62 (2004), pp. 183–85.
59. "New Hepatitis C Virus Screenings Guidelines," last modified August 18, 2012, http://delgadomd.com/hepatitis-c-screening/.
60. Ibid.
61. D. Applebaum et al., "Natural and Traditional Medicine in Cuba: Lessons For U.S. Medical Education." *MEDICC Review* Vol. 10, No. 1 (2008), pp. 43–48.
62. D. Applebaum et al., Natural and Traditional Medicine; Geoff D'Arcy, "Cuba's Green Revolution: the balm to the Achilles heel of Castro's Revolution," *Boletín Latinoamericano y del Caribe de Plantas Medicinales y Aromáticas* Vol. 5, No. 5 (2006), pp. 96–99.

63. N. L. Etkin, "Hausa herbal pharmacopeia. Biomedical evaluation of commonly used plant medicines," *Journal of Ethnopharmacology* 4, (1981): 75–98; Juan Hernández Cano and Gabriele Volpato, "Herbal mixtures in the traditional medicine of Eastern Cuba," *Journal of Ethnopharmacology* Vol. 90, (2004), pp. 293–316; Jesús Guanche, *Procesos Etnoculturales en Cuba,* (Havana: Editorial Letras Cubanas, 1983); Victor Fuentes, "Sobre la medicina tradicional en Cuba: Boletín de Reseña de Plantas Medicinales," *Centro de Información y Documentación Agropecuaria* Vol. 10, (1984), pp. 1-39; M. Rivero de la Calle, "Cuba: A mosaic of races and cultures," (1992), pp. 37–45, quoted in K. Hammer, M. Esquivel, and H. Knu¨pffer, eds., ". . . y tienen faxones y fabas muy diversos de los nuestros. . .," *Evolution and Diversity of Cuban Plant Genetic Resources* Vol. 1; Niurka Núñez González and Estrella González, "Antecedentes etnohistóricos de la alimentación tradicional en Cuba," *Revista Cubana de Alimentación y Nutrición* Vol. 13, (1999), pp. 145–50.
64. Cano and Volpato, "Herbal mixtures in the traditional medicine."
65. Cano and Volpato, op. cit.; D'Arcy, op. cit.
66. Gabrile Volpato, Daimy Godínez, Angela Beyra, and Adelaida Barreto, "Uses of medicinal plants by Haitian immigrants and their descendants in the Province of Camagüey, Cuba," *Journal of Ethnobiology and Ethnomedicine* Vol. 5, No. 16 (2009).
67. D'Arcy, op. cit.
68. Cano and Volpato, op. cit.; Lydia Cabrera, *El Monte* (Havana: Ediciones C.R., 1954); Michel S. Laguerre, *Afro-Caribbean Folk Medicine* (South Hadley, MA: Bergin and Garvey Publishes, Inc., 1987); B.A. Soler and M. Porto, "Experiencia cubana en el estudio y aplicación de medicamentos herbarios," *Revista Cubana de Plantas Medicinales* Vol. 2 (1997), pp. 30–34; Lérida Acosta de la Luz, "Producción de plantas medicinales a pequeña escala: una necesidad de la comunidad," *Revista Cubana de Plantas Medicinales* Vol. 2 (2001), pp. 63–66; D. Applebaum et al., op. cit.
69. World Health Organization, "Legal status of traditional medicine and complementary/alternative medicine: A world wide review" (2001).
70. Pan American Health Organization, "Special Issue on Primary Health Care in the Americas," *Revista Panamericana de Salud Pública* (2007); Félix J. Sansó Sorberats, "Prestar la máxima atención al desarrollo de la medicina natural y tradicional," (2008), pp. 1–8; Martínez Sánchez and Salmon, op. cit.
71. Sansó Sorberats, op. cit.
72. D'Arcy, "Cuba's Green Revolution."
73. D. Applebaum et al., op. cit.
74. Ibid.
75. Ibid.
76. Ibid.
77. Martínez Sánchez and Salmon, op. cit.
78. Ibid.
79. Ministerio de Salud Pública (MINSAP), 1999; Martínez Sánchez and Salmon, op. cit.
80. Martínez Sánchez and Salmon, op. cit.
81. Ibid.
82. Ibid.
83. Juan V. Lorenzo Ginori, "Por una medicina natural y tradicional científica y revolucionaria," speech delivered 2012.
84. Martínez Sánchez and Salmon, "Overview of Complementary/Alternative Medicine."
85. Cano and Volpato, op. cit.; Guanche, op. cit.; Fuentes, op. cit.; Rivero de la Calle, op. cit.; Núñez González and González, op. cit.
86. Cano and Volpato, op. cit.; D. Carbajal et al., "Pharmacological screening of plant decoctions commonly used in Cuban folk medicine," *Journal of Ethnopharmacology* Vol. 33 (1983), pp. 21–24; M.J. Martínez et al., "Screening of some Cuban medicinal plants for antimicrobial activity," *Journal of Ethnopharmacology* Vol. 52, (1996), pp. 171–174; A. Payo, M. Oquendo, and R. Oviedo, "Tamizaje fitoquímico preliminary de

plantas que crecen en Holguín," *Revista Cubana de Farmacia* Vol. 30, No. 2 (1997); M. Guerra, D. Torres, and L. Martínez, "Validación del uso tradicional de plantas medicinales cultivadas en Cuba," *Revista de Plantas Medicinales* Vol. 2, (2001), pp. 48–51.

87. Cano and Volpato, op. cit.

88. Ibid.

89. Ibid.

90. Cano and Volpato, op. cit.; Fuentes, op. cit.

91. J. L. Pérez, R. Miranda, and G. Rodríguez, "Actividad antidepresiva y anticonvulsivante del extracto fluido del *Ocimum tenuiflorum* L.(albahaca morada)," *Revista Cubana de Plantas Medicinales* Vol. 1, (1996), pp. 8–12; J. A. Pino et al., "Composición y propiedades antibacterianas del aceite esencial de *Lippia alba* (Mill.)," *Revista Cubana de Farmacia* Vol. 30, (1997), pp. 1–7; E. Sánchez, I.M. Leal, J. Pino, and C. Carballo, "Estandardización de *Mentha spicata* L. Medicamento herbario con actividad antiespasmódica," *Revista Cubana de Plantas Medicinales* Vol. 3, (1998), pp. 26–30; M. E. Pascual et al., "Lippia: traditional uses, chemistry and pharmacology: a review," *Journal of Ethnopharmacology* Vol. 76, (2001), pp. 201–214; Joane Barnes, Linda A. Anderson, and J. D. Phillipson, *Herbal Medicines: A guide for healthcare professionals (*London: Pharmaceutical Press, 2002); J. T. Roig, *Plantas medicinales, aromáticas o venenosas de Cuba,* (Havana: Ciencia y Técnica, 1974); J. F. Morton, *Atlas of Medicinal Plants of Middle America: Bahamas to Yucatan,* (Springfield, IL: Charles C. Thomas Publisher, 1981); J. Seoane Gallo, *El Folclor Médico de Cuba,* (Havana: Editora Ciencias Sociales, 1984); Victor Fuentes, "Las plantas medicinales en Cuba" (doctoral thesis, La University of Havana, 1988); Emérita Moreno Rodíguez, Mercedes Valero González, and Pedro Pablo Herrera Oliver, "El uso de plantas mágicas y medicinales por las parteras tradicionales cubanas," *Fontqueria* Vol. 39, (1994), pp. 219–241; Cano and Volpato, "Herbal mixtures in the traditional medicine."

92. A. Bachiller, "Cuba primitiva. Origen, lenguas, tradiciones e historiade las indias de las Antillas mayores de Lucayas. Segunda parte,"*Revista de Cuba* Vol. 5, (1879), pp. 26–27; Moreno Rodíguez et al., op. cit.; Cano and Volpato, op. cit.

93. Seoane Gallo, op. cit.; Cano and Volpato, op. cit.

94. Etkin, op. cit.

95. Seoane Gallo, *El Folclor Médico*; A. Aguilar and P. Herrera, "El significado sociocultural de las plantasalimenticias, en las religiones afrocubanas," *Fontqueria* Vol. 42, (1995), pp. 279–87; Moreno Rodíguez et al., op. cit.; Cano and Volpato, op. cit.

96. Etkin, op. cit.

97. K. Vermani and S. Garg, "Herbal medicines for sexually transmitted diseases and AIDS," *Journal of Ethnopharmacology* Vol. 80, (2002), pp. 49–66; Cano and Volpato, op. cit.

98. Cabrera, op. cit.

99. Laguerre, op. cit.; Cano and Volpato, op. cit.

100. T. Johns, *The Origins of Human Diet and Medicine: Chemical Ecology,* (Tucson: University of Arizona Press, 1990); Cano and Volpato, op. cit.

101. Cano and Volpato, "Herbal mixtures in the traditional medicine."

102. B. Weniger, "Interest and limitations of a global ethnopharmacological survey," *Journal of Ethnopharmacology* Vol. 32, (1991), pp. 37–41; Cano and Volpato, op. cit.

103. O.A. Binutu, "Phytochemical and antimicrobial studies on *Crescentia cujete,*" *Fitoterapia* Vol. 68, (1997), pp. 184–85; T. Kaneko, K. Ohtani, R. Kasai, K. Yamasaki, M.D. Nguyen, "Iridoids and iridoid glucosides from fruits ofCrescentia cujete," *Phytochemistry* Vol. 46, (1997), pp. 907–10; Kaneko et al., "*n*-Alkyl glycosides and *p*-hydroxybenzoyloxy glucose from fruits of *Crescentia cujete,*" *Phytochemistry* Vol. 47, (1998), pp. 259–63; Roig, op. cit.; Victor Fuentes and M. Granda, "Estudios sobre la medicina tradicional en Cuba," *Revista de Plantas Medicinales* Vol. 2, (1982), pp. 25–46; Seoane Gallo, op. cit.; Moreno Rodíguez et al., op. cit.; Cano and Volpato, op. cit.

104. F. Ortiz, *La cocina afrocubana,* in *Gusta Usted?*, (La Havana: Imprenta Oscar Garcia S.A., 1956); Gabriele Volpato and Daimy Godínez, "Ethnobotany of *pru,* a tradition-

al Cuban refreshment," *Journal of Economic Botany* Vol. 58, (2004), pp. 381–95; Cano and Volpato, op. cit.

105. Volpato and Godínez, op. cit.; Cano and Volpato, op. cit.

106. "Traditional Medicine: Definitions," http://www.who.int/medicines/areas/traditional/definitions/en/ .

107. Winsome B. Christie, "Herbs safety in use"(paper presented at CARPIN 3rd Scientific Conference, Kingston, Jamaica, May 31–June 1, 2008); Cano and Volpato, op. cit.; K. Chan, "Some aspects of toxic contaminants in herbal medicine," *Chemosphere* Vol. 52 (2003), pp. 1361–371; Jennifer H.A. Paul and Compton E. Seaforth, "Harmful plants in Caribbean folk medicine," *Focus on Alternative and Complementary Therapies,* Special Issue: Caribbean Herbal Medicine, Vol. 16 (2011), pp. 261–5.

108. Cano and Volpato, op. cit.; K. Chan, op. cit.; Jennifer H.A. Paul and Compton E. Seaforth, "Harmful plants in Caribbean Folk Medicine." *Focus on Alternative and Complementary Therapies* Vol. 16 (2011), pp. 261–65.

109. Jennifer Kelly, "Toxicity and Adverse Effects of Herbal Complimentary Therapy," *NursingTimes.net,* May 1, 2002; P. F. D'Arcy "Adverse reactions and interactions with herbal medicines. Part 1–Adverse reactions." *Adverse Drug React Toxicol Rev,* Vol. 10, No. 4 (Winter 1991), pp. 189–208; P. F. D'Arcy, "Adverse reactions and interactions with herbal medicines. Part 2–Drug interactions," *Adverse Drug React Toxicol Rev,* Vol. 12, No. 3 (1993 Autumn), pp. 147–162; A. Vickers and C. Zollman, "ABC of complementary medicine: herbal medicine," *BMJ* Vol. 319 (1999), pp. 1050–1053.

110. Cano and Volpato, op. cit.

111. Chan, op. cit.

112. Christie, op. cit.

113. Binutu, "Phytochemical and antimicrobial studies"; Kaneko et al., "Iridoids and iridoid glucosides"; Kaneko et al., "*n*-Alkyl glycosides and *p*-hydroxybenzoyloxy glucose"; Roig, op. cit.; Fuentes and Granda, op. cit.; Gallo, op. cit.; Rodíguez et al., op. cit.; Cano and Volpato, op. cit.

SEVEN

Medical Diplomacy, Medical Services

In 1960 Cuba was suffering from an exodus of medical professionals and significant economic losses from not only the aftermath of war but prolonged battles with insurgents in the Escambray Mountains.[1] That same year the most powerful earthquake ever recorded struck southern Chile, killing thousands and causing massive landslides, flooding, and a series of tsunamis that battered the South American nation's coast.[2] The Great Valdivia Earthquake drew the world's attention to a rather isolated corner of the world and the Castro government, despite its limited resources, decided to send a small medical team to Chile, its first of many medical missions abroad.

Jorge Alessandri, Chile's president at the time, was a conservative with little sympathy for the Cuban revolution, but two years later Chile would abstain during a vote for a U.S.-backed resolution in the Organization of American States to exclude Cuba. Chile maintained diplomatic relations until 1964, reestablished ties during the socialist government of Salvador Allende, breaking relations after the 1973 military coup and then moving to a limited relationship at the consular level in 1991, a year after a democratically elected government took office. Full diplomatic relations were restored in 1995, and once again, Cuban medical diplomacy played a role.

In 1990 the two-year-old son of a conservative Chilean politician, Andres Allamand, suffered severe neurological damage after nearly drowning in a swimming pool. A few months later the family was approached, through intermediaries, by the Castro government, which offered to treat the child at a neurosurgery center in Havana. The Centro Internacional de Restauración Neurológica (CIREN) had just opened the previous year, and according to Allamand, the invitation came directly from Fidel Castro himself.

"I will never forget the way he helped us with my son's recuperation," Allamand later told an interviewer. "I have always separated the political plane of my vision of the Cuban dictatorship from the human gestures Fidel Castro made toward my son Juan Andres."[3] According to Allamand, Castro took a personal interest in the case from the time of the family's arrival, participating in discussions among medical staff as if he were a doctor and making multiple visits to the child's bedside.[4]

Cuban medical staff accompanied the family when they returned to Santiago, and Castro telephoned several times to inquire about the child's progress. Several years later when Juan Andres died, the Chilean politician and his wife decided to scatter his ashes in Cuba.[5] It is not clear whether the Cuban government or the Allamand family paid for the child's treatment and the family's travel expenses, at a time when the Cuban economy was reeling from the loss of Soviet subsidies and aid, and there were no details of the nature of the medical treatment received or whether it was something unavailable in Chile. But the conservative Chilean politician became a proponent of closer ties with Cuba, and at one point contacted one of Castro's aides to request a Cuban-produced medication on behalf of a friend. The unidentified medication, supposedly available only in Cuba, arrived in Santiago within days.[6]

Some critics viewed the Allamand case as the cynical manipulation of a vulnerable family, but whatever Castro's true motives, this and other instances of medical diplomacy have earned Cuba considerable goodwill and increasingly, economic benefits. Since coming to power the Castro government has sent Cuban physicians to over 100 countries as emergency medical assistance and more extended health projects. The mission to Chile was followed by a longer engagement in Algeria, with a team of twenty-nine doctors, fifteen nurses, three dentists, and eight medical technicians, who landed in the country on May 24, 1963, accompanied by Cuba's then-Minister for Public Health, Jose Ramon Machado Ventura. The group had been given no language training, only a brief lecture at the Cuban foreign ministry, where the official in charge of North Africa told them Algeria was a tropical country and they should pack short-sleeved shirts. They were not issued passports, but sheets of paper from the foreign ministry, and were not told how long they would be in Algeria.

Upon arrival, the Cuban medical team found the weather much colder and Machado Ventura had to buy them overcoats. After a week in Algiers, the Cuban medical professionals were divided up and sent to hospitals in different Algerian towns. Algeria provided accommodation, but the Cubans had no access to food other than what was served at the hospital canteens, while officials from both countries worked out who would pay for the Cubans' living expenses.[7]

The Algerian project was part of the Castro government's support for anticolonial movements in Africa, and the services of Cuban health professionals were usually an adjunct to military aid. In the mid-1970s, Cuba launched a massive military intervention to support the leftist People's Movement for the Liberation of Angola, and teams of Cuban medical personnel accompanied thousands of Cuban troops. Cuban doctors and other health care personnel began working in clinics and hospitals throughout most of the country, and continue working in Angola today.

Cuba has also sent medical relief teams to assist earthquake victims in Peru in 1970 and Nicaragua in 1972, and to hurricane victims in Honduras in 1974 and 1998. But some offers of medical aid have been more political showmanship than humanitarian. On August 30, 2005, Fidel Castro publicly offered to send 1,000 Cuban doctors to work in areas of the United States devastated by Hurricane Katrina. There was no response from the Bush administration, but in a televised speech Castro announced he had raised the number of would be medical volunteers to 1,586, with another 300 in reserve, and named the group the Henry Reeve Brigade, after an American who had joined Cuba's fight for independence from Spain.

Photographs showed doctors seated with green camouflage backpacks in their laps during the Castro speech. According to MEDICC, the Cuban health professionals were committed to remaining in the disaster areas as long as needed and included "specialists in family medicine, cardiology, pediatrics, epidemiology and other fields, and trained in disaster response and health risks engendered by such events, the health professionals were outfitted with two backpacks each, filled with 24 kilograms (52.8 pounds) of essential medicines." The backpacks also contained "re-hydration therapies, insulin, hypertension medications, treatments for systemic and topical infections, and minor surgical instruments."[8] If this is an accurate account, one wonders how such supplies were gathered so quickly when Cuba's own medical facilities were suffering from shortages.

It is interesting to compare Castro's offer of aid to Katrina victims with the response of Doctors Without Borders/Médecins San Frontiéres (MSF). Other than a small support program for 9/11 responders, the organization shared the same lack of experience in the United States as Cuba's Henry Reeve Brigade and thus had "limited logistical capacity and expertise."[9] On September 2 a five-member assessment team experienced in emergency relief work toured the Gulf areas affected by the disaster, meeting with Red Cross and other relief organizations to determine how MSF might contribute to the relief efforts. The assessment team's conclusion was that "there was a capacity to evacuate people in urgent need of medical care, so there was not a great need for our help" and that "it does not look like MSF has a role to play in providing assistance to the victims of Hurricane Katrina."[10]

Cuba's international medical missions have not always made the best use of health care professionals' time and training. In the absence of medical facilities and pharmacies, Cuban doctors sent to remote areas are unable to make full use of their abilities and risk a deterioration in their professional skills as a result. Many find themselves performing a role closer to that of a social worker. One physician was posted to the Brazilian interior in the late 1990s "without a word of Portuguese" and once he managed to learn enough of the language to communicate with local people he emphasized diet and lifestyle changes in his dealings with the local community. The lack of any clinical resources in the area made it difficult to actually treat patients.[11]

Dr. Eloy Gonzalez, an oncologist, was sent to Nicaragua in 1987, only to learn upon his arrival that the program did not require a cancer specialist. He and nine other doctors met with the deputy chief of the Cuban mission, who when informed of Gonzalez's medical background, left the room for several minutes and returned to inform him that from now on he was to work as a specialist in internal medicine.[12]

Dr. Leonel Cordova, who volunteered for a program in Zimbabwe in 2000, was assigned to a Harare hospital, but was prevented from working due to the Zimbabwe medical association's objections to the Cuban doctors. The issue was not resolved for approximately six months, and he and his colleagues were left in a hotel with nothing to do in the meantime.[13]

Cuba's most extensive international health project was with Venezuela, where as many as 40,000 doctors and other health professionals have worked. The first accord was signed in 2000, the year after Hugo Chavez became president, and provided subsidized Venezuelan oil to Cuba in exchange for the services of Cuban health teams, engineers, and teachers. There would be a network of community health clinics in poor and underserved communities in the program known as Barrio Adentro, with 8,500 primary care facilities constructed around the country by the end of 2004. But by May 2007 only 2,708 modules had been built, at a cost of US$126.5 million funded by the Venezuelan state petroleum company, with another 3,284 under construction.[14]

Of those community health facilities that had been built, an estimated 30 percent were empty, which Venezuelan health officials attributed to a continuing shortage of doctors. Adolfo Delgado, head of the Venezuelan Bolivarian Society of General Integral Medicine, told the British medical journal *The Lancet* that the personnel shortage could be eased by allowing medical students, who were then working as assistants to Barrio Adentro doctors, to work alone in treating patients.[15]

While many Cuban doctors felt proud of their role in delivering care to the poor, conditions in the Barrio Adentro program were often harsh and extremely dangerous. Venezuela has one of the world's highest murder rates, and living and working in poor communities left them exposed to the same dangers as local residents. Neither government has revealed any figures for those assaulted, raped, or killed, but in 2010 a ceremony was held in Caracas honoring sixty-eight Cuban health professionals who had died in the country.[16] Doctors in the program received free accommodation, and the monthly pay was ten times the $20–25 typically received at home, but hardly enough to cover their expenses. Their families back in Cuba received the doctors' usual monthly income plus bonuses and money deposited in a reserve fund that is made available upon their return. As another economic incentive, Cuban health personnel were allowed to send home three large boxes of goods per year, with no shipping costs or import taxes to be paid. One Cuban physician who worked in Venezuela from 2006 to 2009 said his family received $50 per month the first two years he was abroad, which increased to $100 after that. He forfeited his accumulated reserve fund, worth about $2,000, when he defected.[17]

Cuban health personnel working in Venezuela are restricted in their movements and kept under close watch by police and intelligence groups, but some still manage to break away and seek political asylum. There are no exact figures on the number of Cuban health personnel who sought political asylum while working in Venezuela, but according to Solidaridad Sin Fronteras, a Miami organizations that assists Cuban medical professionals, around 3,000arrived from Venezuela in 2013, a 60 percent increase over the previous year.[18] A confidential cable from the U.S. Embassy in Caracas reported that from August 2006 to April 2009 it had received 739 requests for asylum from Cuban medical professionals working in Venezuela. The cable also quotes a Venezuelan academic who said that while the Barrio Adentro program had not improved health outcomes, "even if the doctors were not the most professionally capable, they were able to attend to common medical problems, dispense aspirin, and provide psychological reassurance that boosted Barrio residents' morale and Chavez's popularity." The cable noted in its summary that although "plagued by mismanagement, corruption and inefficiency, Barrio Adentro nevertheless has improved access to medical services for some of Venezuela's poor, albeit without eliminating or even alleviating long-term problems in the health care system."[19]

The Chavez government also expanded medical education programs and announced that Venezuela would open a branch of Cuba's Latin American School of Medicine (ELAM) in the southern state of Bolivar. Chavez broadcast one of his television programs, Alo Presidente, from the school's planned site and announced that the facility would initially train 500 students from Latin American countries, with an eventual capacity for 1,920 students. There would be twenty-eight classrooms and two auditoriums, he said.[20] The school was never completed, though a number of Cuban physicians worked in Venezuela's expanded medical schools.

On December 23, 2009, Chavez announced a new Cuban-Venezuelan initiative aimed at lowering maternal and infant mortality rates. "Operation Baby Jesus" would provide healthy nutrition for women of child-bearing age, especially for pregnant women, and newborn babies. Breastfeeding would be encouraged, and there would be a special focus on the health of children under five, with measures to detect any physical and mental disabilities. He made the announcement on television, while inaugurating a new intensive neonatal unit at a general hospital on the outskirts of Caracas, and said $150 million would be spent on the first stage of the project to improve obstetric services in Venezuelan hospitals and to build temporary prenatal residences for women with high risk pregnancies.[21] It is not clear what impact this and other Cuba-supported health programs had on maternal-infant health, but the country's infant mortality rate in 2000 had been 26.17 per 1,000 births, dropping to 22.2 in 2005, then 21.07 in 2010. The available figures for maternal mortality suggest either no change or a slight deterioration, from 91 deaths per 100,000 births in 2000, increasing to 94 in 2005 and dropping to 92 in 2010.[22] As mentioned in chapter 3, Cuba's own official health statistics show lowered rates of infant mortality alongside significantly higher rates of maternal mortality, two health indicators which usually improve at the same time. Venezuelan authorities did not publish health statistics after 2010.

The Chavez government also funded Cuban health missions in other developing countries, particularly in those with avowedly leftist governments such as Nicaragua, Bolivia, and Ecuador. Shortly after the election of Evo Morales, Bolivia's first indigenous president, over 700 Cuban doctors arrived in the country, and by April of 2008 there were 1,226 physicians along with 626 nurses and other health care personnel. The Cuban presence sparked protests in both Venezuela and Bolivia, with local doctors complaining that many of the Cubans did not hold proper medical qualifications and were undermining their efforts to negotiate salaries and better working conditions.[23]

Another project was "Operation Miracle," launched in 2004 to provide eye surgery, mostly cataract operations, by bringing patients to Cuba or else setting up eye clinics in other countries. Venezuelans were the first beneficiaries of the program, with many treated at Havana's Hermanos Almeijeiras Hospital. The facility, which was featured in Michael Moore's documentary Sicko, has two floors reserved for foreigners. A U.S. Foreign Service medical officer visited in 2007 and was told that Venezuelan patients received a weekly toiletry kit of Colgate toothpaste, Palmolive soap, and Palmolive shampoo, and that they "frequently take these items outside to the front parking lot and sell them to local Cubans." Cuban patients received the toothpaste and no other toiletries.[24]

Additional eye surgical clinics were built in Venezuela, and both countries began to receive foreign patients under the program. The director of the Paraguayan Health Ministry's Program for Ocular Health, Dr. Luz Marina Quintana, told U.S. Embassy officials in Asuncion that the surgeries performed in Venezuela were "substantially better" than those performed in Cuba, but that the Paraguayan patients received inadequate follow-up care.[25]

Under normal circumstances most patients undergoing eye surgeries such as cataract operations do not require hospitalization, and need only wear eye protection, apply prescribed eye drops at regular intervals, and attend a series of follow-up visits to their ophthalmologist. Flying patients to Havana or Caracas and interning them in hospitals or other accommodation seems wasteful, and some of the passengers aboard the chartered flights were not patients at all but going for "community leadership training."[26] In one strange incident, a group of 163 Paraguayans remained in Cuba for an entire month before they were flown home; a Paraguayan health ministry official said that Cuban authorities had indicated there would be a "recess" in the chartered flights taking Paraguayans to the island and that the Paraguayan government was undertaking a "technical evaluation" of the program.[27]

During this period Venezuela's own public health system suffered from neglect and poor coordination with the Barrio Adentro program. In theory the Cuba-staffed facilities were supposed to provide primary care in underserved communities, but many Venezuelans did not make use of them and persisted in seeking basic medical care from hospitals. A second stage of the program in 2005 opened dozens of new, high tech facilities for diagnostics, rehabilitation, and other services rather than invest and expand in existing hospitals. The next year saw the opening of around 300 more new high tech centers, while falling short of a stated goal to build 1,235 more primary care facilities in poor Venezuelan neighborhoods.[28]

The deterioration in Venezuela's public health facilities seemed to accelerate after Chavez's death from cancer on March 5, 2013, even as his successor, Nicolas Maduro, promised there would be no change in Chavez's political project or the country's tight relationship with Cuba. According to the Venezuelan Medical Federation, half the public health system's doctors resigned during the Chavez government and half of those left the country. Both public and private hospitals suffered shortages of supplies and broken equipment, while staff departures at the Caracas blood bank meant that donations could only be taken on weekday mornings.[29]

In addition to Venezuela, Cuba has other sources of financial backing for medical missions in other countries. In 2004, South Africa signed a $1 million agreement to finance Cuban health projects in other African countries, with a team of over 100 Cuban doctors going to Mali. In 2010, South Africa agreed to fund thirty-one Cuban medical professionals working in Rwanda.[30] Additional funds have come from the Pan American Health Organization (PAHO) and Japan and some European countries have provided financing for Cuban missions in Honduras. After Hurricane Mitch ravaged the Central American country in 2005,

Germany, France, and Japan worked with PAHO to provide $400 per month for each Cuban doctor sent to Honduras, along with medicines.[31]

Haiti's 2010 earthquake seemed to draw world attention to the work of Cuban medical missions abroad and generated a large amount of favorable publicity. Cuban doctors had been working in the country since 1996 and in 1998 the two countries signed a bilateral agreement covering health cooperation, education, tourism, sports, and agriculture. The accord also provided specialized medical training for 100 Haitian doctors at Cuban hospitals, and Haitian students would later be among the first class enrolled at the Latin American Medical School when it opened its doors. There was also a project in which France provided funds for Cuban vaccination programs and HIV/AIDS projects in the country; according to one Cuban doctor who worked in Haiti from 2002 to 2003 the program in which he worked had been funded entirely by France.[32]

There were 344 Cuban health professionals in Haiti at the time of the earthquake and their numbers had declined from 579 in 2004 as the Castro government began to send more and more people to Venezuela. Despite the fact that the Cubans were spread out among 127 of Haiti's municipalities, official reports said they had performed 1,000 emergency surgeries within the first twenty-four hours.[33] Cuba sent a contingent from its Henry Reeve Brigade within twenty-four hours, and according to MEDICC, this group was formed of a carefully selected team of "surgeons, orthopaedists, dermatologists epidemiologists, psychologists, nurses and obstetricians."[34]

The most pressing need, however, would have been for experienced orthopedic surgeons and traumatologists to treat the many crush injuries victims suffered from collapsing buildings and falling debris. Only ten days after the earthquake, Cuban medical personnel reportedly carried out 1,054 surgeries and over the first twenty-eight days following the disaster performed 3,400 surgeries, the Cuban government press reported.[35] According to Anthony Redmond, a British doctor and professor of international emergency medicine who studied international medical relief efforts in Haiti during this period, many Haitians were subjected to unnecessary amputations by doctors with insufficient experience in orthopedic injuries. He concluded from his findings that amputation rates for people with crushed limbs varied from 5 percent to 45 percent of patients, and that those treated by smaller and less experienced medical teams were more likely to have arms and legs amputated than those treated by physicians working for large charities.[36] Redmond declined to reveal the amputation rates for Cuban medical teams or any of the other relief groups working in Haiti, saying he had given his word "to all those who allowed me to review their data from their work in Haiti that I would not identify the amputation rates of any specific team."[37]

It is not clear how long the Cuban emergency medical brigade remained in Haiti, and some of the numbers cited include Haitian graduates of ELAM, ELAM students, and nonmedical personnel. In October of that year Haiti suffered an outbreak of cholera, and Cuba sent another contingent of 300 health care professionals to fight the epidemic. Norway provided $850,000 for the anticholera program, and it is not clear how much of this was spent on medications and supplies, or Cuban salaries.[38]

Brazil has also given financial support to Cuban medical projects in Haiti, and this relationship gave way to a controversial agreement to bring thousands of Cuban doctors to work in poor and underserved Brazilian communities. In June of 2013 the country was rocked by mass demonstrations protesting poor public transportation, education, and health services. Brazil has 1.8 physicians per 1,000 people, one of the lowest among countries who are members of the Organization for Economic Cooperation and Development. The government of Dilma Rousseff soon announced Brazil would hire up to 6,000 foreign doctors, mostly Cubans, in a program known as Mais Medicos (More Doctors). The Pan American Health Organization would help manage the program, which paid $4,255 per month per doctor, with the doctors themselves receiving only a portion of this and an undisclosed amount going to the Cuban government, which badly needed new sources of revenue.

The announcement drew immediate fire from much of Brazil's medical community. The Cuban doctors would not have to pass the Brazilian government's medical qualifying examinations in order to practice, and Brazilian physicians, noting the high failure rate among Cuban-trained doctors (see chapter 5), questioned the Cubans' qualifications for treating their country's most vulnerable patients. Dr. Jose Bonamigo, director of the Brazilian Medical Association, pointed out Cuban doctors' unfamiliarity with the much broader range of primary care medications used in Brazil, which could cause complications for patients. He observed that primary care physicians in Cuba had access to only ten to fifteen commonly prescribed drugs.

The association had not been invited to take part in discussions about Brazil's physician shortage with the government prior to the announcement. Bonamigo noted that Brazilian officials had stated that the Cuban and other foreign doctors working in remote areas would be provided with the supplies and medications needed, but that based on the past experiences of Brazilian medical personnel in the country's outlying regions, the outlook was not good.[39]

In an open letter the association said the Mais Medicos program disguised the real problems afflicting Brazil's public health system, including a neglected infrastructure and lack of beds, ambulances, and medications. "It is the lack of investment and the incompetent management of this system that drives away Brazilian doctors," the letter said.[40]

The Rousseff government responded that Cuban doctors would be working in primary care settings and in only those posts where no Brazilian doctors were available, would not be performing surgery or other specialist work and would be closely supervised. The Justice Ministry would accept applications for political asylum, though no Cubans had done so during the first few months of the program. The Brazilian public seemed to support the program; one poll showed that 84.3 percent of those queried were in favor, although a smaller majority—66 percent—thought the foreign doctors were qualified to work in the country. The first group of Cuban doctors to arrive in Brazil landed at the Fortaleza Airport in northeastern Brazil, and were confronted by angry local doctors shouting "Slaves!" at them. The scene was filmed by an onlooker and posted on the Internet, and the sight of the Cubans walking slowly and quietly past the jeering protestors may have improved the program's image further.

Within a few months, however, some of the newly arrived Cuban physicians began leaving their posts. Dr. Ramona Rodriguez arrived in Brazil in October 2013 and was assigned to a municipality in the northeastern state of Pará in the country's northeast Amazon region. A few months later she sought refuge in the office of a local center-right politician, and gave a speech to the Brazilian congress in which she accused the Rousseff government of treating Cuban doctors "like slave labor." She held up a copy of Pan American Health Organization contract and said that the Cuban government took too big a chunk of her pay. According to the terms of the contract, Cuban doctors were to receive only one fifth of the approximately US$4,200 monthly payment Brazil was paying for each doctor, with the rest going to the Cuban state.[41]

When a second Cuban doctor defected, Brazil's health minister, Arthur Chioro, held a press conference to announce that Cuban physicians would have their wages raised. This did not entail Brazil paying more, but negotiations with PAHO and the Cuban government had produced an agreement in which Cuba would pay $1,000 a month directly to the doctors and another $245 to be deposited in an account in Cuba, he said.[42]

Brazil's former health minister, Alexandre Padilha, predicted the Cuban doctors would make a contribution to easing his country's shortage of physicians. "It's easier and quicker to train a doctor to fluently speak Portuguese than wait six years for them to graduate," he said. Padilha recalled his own experience working in indigenous communities in the Brazilian Amazon region, saying "I saved lots of Indian lives and I don't speak any indigenous languages."[43]

Some of the Cuban doctors did encounter health conditions for which they had no experience. One doctor, speaking in a mixture of Portuguese and Spanish, told the Reuters news agency that she had come across "illnesses here that I had only read about in books, like leprosy, which no longer exists in Cuba."[44] But the program continued to earn praise from poor Brazilians (as well as boost the Rousseff government's poll numbers.)

The Mais Medicos was one of the most lucrative for the Cuban government, one of a growing number of medical services contracts it has signed with other governments. In July 2013, Cuba and Saudi Arabia reached a deal to provide physicians to the kingdom's Visiting Doctors program, which brings in foreign specialists for temporary assignments in Saudi hospitals. Under this program, thirty Cuban doctors would arrive every three months, replacing Cuban medical teams completing their postings. There was no word on how much the Cuban physicians or the Cuban government would be paid.[45] Cuba also has a medical services agreement with Yemen, but neither government has revealed any details. A Yemeni news agency reported a meeting between the Cuban ambassador and the country's minister for public health and population, with the former "pointing out the fruitful results carried out by Cuban medical teams for Yemen."[46]

Ecuador signed an agreement for the provision of 1,000 Cuban doctors, mostly primary care physicians to work in the country beginning in 2014. The program will cost $30 million annually, according to President Rafael Correa.[47] At least twenty other countries have medical service contracts with Cuba, and while the Castro government does not publish figures on the total value of these health service exports, the category of "services" in Cuba's annual export figures has increased from 6.6 billion pesos in 2006 to 10.8 billion pesos in 2011.[48]

NOTES

1. Fighting by pro-Batista soldiers and former guerrillas who had broken with Castro lasted until 1965 and was named the War against the Bandits by the Castro government.
2. Estimates of the number killed and injured vary; according to data from the Center for Research on the Epidemiology of Disasters database, 6,000 were killed, http://www.emdat.be/result-country-profile
3. *La Nacion*, January 16, 2013.
4. *El Mercurio*, July 11, 2006. The director of CIREN, Dr. Hilda Molina, resigned in protest in 1994 over a government directive to reserve places at the hospital for foreign patients.
5. Ibid.
6. *Revista Capital*, January 23, 2011.
7. Piero Gleijeses, "Cuba's First Venture in Africa: Algeria 1961–65," *Journal of Latin American Studies*, Vol. 28, No. 1 (February, 1996), pp. 159–96.
8. Connor Gorry, "Cuba's Response to Katrina Disaster," *MEDICC Review*, Vol. 7, No. 8 (August-September 2005).
9. "Hurricane Katrina: MSF's Exploratory Mission to Louisiana," September 6, 2005, http://www.doctorswithoutborders.org/news/article.cfm?id=1579
10. Ibid
11. Joe Leahy, "Cuban doctors bring "quick fix" to Brazil's vast remote interior," *Financial Times*, December 23, 2013.
12. Interview with Dr. Eloy Gonzalez, December 13, 2013.
13. Interview with Dr. Leonel Cordova, August 14, 2013. He and a Cuban colleague tried to seek asylum at the United Nations High Commission for Refugees, but were

arrested and placed on a flight to Johannesburg, with a scheduled connections to Paris and Havana. The two sought help from Air France crew members, who refused to put them and their security guards on the flight, and South African authorities sent them back to Harare. Cordova and his colleague later received asylum in the United States.

14. Rachel Jones, "Hugo Chavez' health-care program misses its goals," *The Lancet*, June 14, 2008.

15. Ibid.

16. Maria Werlau, "Cuba-Venezuela Health Diplomacy: the Business of Humanitarianism," Cuba in Transition, Association for the Study of the Cuban Economy, 2010.

17. Ibid.

18. "En un año tres mil cubanos desertaron de Venezuela," *Cubanet*, December 21, 2013.

19. "Barrio Adentro crisis: Chavez to strengthen flagship medical program in advance of elections," classified State Department cable from the U.S. Embassy in Caracas, October 26, 2009. Released by Wikileaks, https://www.wikileaks.org/plusd/cables/09CARACAS1374_a.html

20. Ministerio de Comunicación e Información, "Develada piedra fundacional de la Escuela Latinoamericana de Medicina en Pueblo Guri," May 22, 2006, http://www.aporrea.org/educacion/n78010.html

21. Tamara Pearson, "New Venezuelan Mission Aims to Lower Maternal and Infant Mortality Rates," *Venezuelanalysis*, December 24, 2009.

22. WHO, UNICEF, UNFPA, World Bank and UN Population Division Maternal Mortality Estimation Inter-Agency Group.

23. BBC, "Venezuela medics march over jobs," July 15, 2005; and BBC, "Bolivia protest over Cuba medics," June 22, 2006.

24. "Cuban Health Care: "Aqui nada es facil" (Here nothing is easy), classified State Department cable from the U.S. Interests Section in Havana dated January 31, 2008 and released by Wikileaks, http://www.wikileaks.org/plusd/cables/08HAVANA103_a.html

25. "Venezuelans Performing Eye Surgeries and More," confidential US Embassy cable from Asuncion dated October 24, 2008 and released by Wikileaks, http://www.wikileaks.org/plusd/cables/08ASUNCION720_a.html

26. The Paraguayan newspaper ABC Color reported that the program had been extended without any consultation with the country's Health Ministry, and that each of the Venezuelan-chartered flights transported 30-50 Paraguayans travelling for "community leadership" training. See Gonzalez Vera, Roque, "Nadie sabe lo que hacen los jovenes en Venezuela," ABC Color, Octover 12, 2008.

27. "Luego de casi un mes, llegan Paraguayos que fueron a Cuba," ABC Color, December 7, 2005.

28. Daniel Cancel, "In Venezuela, two public-health systems grow apart." *The Lancet*, August 11, 2007.

29. Frank Bajak, "Doctors say Venezuela's Health Care in Collapse," *New York Times*, November 6, 2013.

30. Julie Feinsilver, "Fifty Years of Cuba's Medical Diplomacy: From Idealism to Pragmatism," *Cuban Studies*, Vol. 41 (2010).

31. Maria Werlau, "Cuba's Business of Humanitarianism: The Medical Mission in Haiti," Association for the Study of the Cuban Economy, Cuba in Transition, 2011.

32. Ibid.

33. John Burnett, "Cuban doctors unsung heroes of Haitian earthquake," National Public Radio broadcast, January 24, 2010.

34. Connor Gorry, "Once the Earth Stood Still (Part 1): Cuban Rehabilitative Services in Haiti," *MEDICC Review*, Vol. 12, No. 2 (Spring 2010), http://www.medicc.org/mediccreview/index.php?issue=12&id=145&a=vahtml.

35. Werlau, op cit.

36. Hannah Devlin, "Disaster tourist docs too quick to amputate," *The Times*, June 4, 2013.

37. Interview with Dr. Anthony Redmond, August 6, 2013.
38. Werlau, op cit.
39. Interview with Dr. Jose Bonamigo, July 10, 2013.
40. Associacao Medica Brasileira, Carta aberta aos médicos e à população brasileira, June 22, 2013, http://www.amb.org.br/Site/Home/NOT%C3%8DCIAS/Carta-aberta-aos-m%C3%A9dicos-e-%C3%A0-popula%C3%A7%C3%A3o-brasileira%2036892.cnt.
41. Anthony Boadle, "Cuban doctor defects in Brazil over pay, seeks asylum," *Reuters*, February 5, 2014.
42. Matthew Cowley, "Cuba to Raise Pay of Doctors Working in Brazil," *Wall Street Journal*, February 28, 2014; and EFE, "Pay raise for Cuban doctors recruited by Brazil," February 28, 2014.
43. Goodman, Joshua, "Castro Doctors Help Brazil Ease Shortage as Rules Relaxed," Bloomberg, September 20, 2013.
44. Anthony Boadle, "Cuban doctors tend to Brazil's poor, giving Rousseff a boost," *Reuters*, December 1, 2012.
45. Rasooldeen, MD, "Team of specialized Cuban doctors arriving to man hospitals," Arabnews.com, August 3, 2013.
46. "Yemen, Cuba discuss cooperation in medical area," *Sabanet*, November 19, 2013.
47. "Cuban doctors to arrive in Ecuador in December," *Cuba Standard*, November 21, 2013.
48. Anuario Estadistico de Cuba 2011.

Conclusions: Facing the Future

Shortly before Christmas 2013, heavy rains hit the Cuban capital, causing over 200 buildings to collapse and forcing 2,240 people to be evacuated. According to official figures, 39 percent of the country's housing stock is in poor condition; other estimates put the figure at 57 percent.[1] Dwellings in Old Havana were among the most affected, and the historic section of the city has attracted approximately 80,000 unregistered migrants from other parts of the country, drawn by the tourist industry and the municipality has "some population areas of great social indiscipline."[2]

With increased urbanization comes an increased risk of communicable diseases, and Old Havana has a female HIV/AIDS rate of 11.1 per 10,000 inhabitants—a low infection level compared to many countries, but one which represents the highest among women in Cuba and one which has increased sevenfold since 1986.[3] There have also been recent increases in the incidence of asthma, cholera, diarrhea, hepatitis, TB, and certain vector-borne diseases which are likely a reflection of socioeconomic stress and environmental factors, as well as the weakening of the public health infrastructure. The increase in the incidence of asthma in the population has been of special concern and appears to be a direct result of a decline in housing conditions in the country, increased pollution, and a lack of pharmaceuticals to treat the associated ailments.

In the southeastern municipality of San Miguel del Padron, health workers reported an outbreak of hepatitis A, caused by contaminated food and water, with at least seventy-six cases noted in March 2014. A doctor at a local polyclinic observed that area sewage and waterworks were in bad condition, and that she and her colleagues were expecting the number of cases to rise.[4]

Sometimes patients go without treatment for reasons of simple bureaucratic inertia. A group of eighty cancer patients at the Almejeiras Hospital in the adjacent municipality of Centro Habana went without radiation therapy for two months because of equipment breakdown. MINSAP purchased a linear accelerator for an inoperative ionizing radiation machine, which finally arrived in the Cuban capital on December 16, 2013 but no one bothered to pick it up until three weeks later.[5]

In western Havana lies the more affluent municipality of Miramar where the Clinica Central Cira Garcia is located. Canadians and Europeans visit the facility for such procedures as knee replacement surgery or cosmetic procedures and Latin Americans from countries with restrictive abortion laws undertake the procedure there. The clinic and others catering to foreigners seem to be flourishing, and might even be overwhelmed with a flood of paying customers when U.S. travel and trade sanctions are lifted.[6] One can only speculate what Cubans, frustrated by long waits and the shortages of basic medical supplies in their own public health facilities, must think of such arrangements. P. Sean Brotherton describes helping a Cuban woman purchase a medication from one of the "foreigners" pharmacies that was unavailable in the public pharmacies serving Cubans. He quotes her as saying, "In this country, *los extranjeros* [foreigners] come first. *El pueblo* [locals], on the other hand, we eat shit."[7] In another incident, he accompanies a Cuban friend, whose job as a newspaper editor required good vision and who had been waiting for months for a pair of subsidized eyeglasses from his local clinic, to an optician in Miramar operated by the government's health tourism department, Servimed. For $76, the equivalent of several months' salary, his friend could have the needed gas permeable lenses in three days, with a three-year warranty.[8]

One worst case scenario for the future involves an increasing expansion of health tourism in Cuba which drains some of the best physicians and other professionals away from the public health sector. Medical tourism seems likely to grow, buoyed in part by the country's reputation in health provision and the government's need for additional sources of foreign exchange. In 2011, Cuba launched the Empresa Comercializadora de Servicios Médicos de Cuba S.A., or Servimed, a state holding company to oversee the country's sixteen facilities offering medical services to paying foreign visitors as well as medical contracts to provide health services to other countries. At the same time, Cuba is competing with many other countries for health tourist revenues, including Mexico, India and Brazil and its image could suffer in the post-Castro period when a freer flow of information yields more accounts of medical neglect, malpractice, and mismanagement—dramatic contrasts to the Cuban health sector's carefully protected representation during the Castro period. In short, Cuban health care may suffer from a credibility problem.

According to Dr. Hilda Molina, who was allowed to leave the country in 2009, the hospitals catering to foreigners often advertise services they do not have the resources to perform and are incapable of guaranteeing any better results than what the patients might expect in their own countries. In addition, patients are sometimes given false medical information and steered toward services they do not need.[9]

One of the medical services offered to health tourists has already come under critical scrutiny by international specialists. Retinitis pigmentosa is an inherited eye disease which can lead to vision impairment and blindness, and although there is no cure, the disease's progress can be delayed in some cases by high doses of vitamin A. Since 1992 Cuba has been offering a treatment combining surgery, ozone therapy, vitamin therapy, and electrostimulation, which according to Servimed's website stops the disease's progress in 78 percent of patients.[10] But the program, which charges over $10,000 for a three-week hospital stay plus at least $4,900 for follow up treatments every six months, has not been subjected to any peer review or evaluated by independent medical researchers. Follow up studies in Norway, Germany, and the United States of patients who had undergone the Cuban treatment failed to document any improvements in vision, and in some cases even worsened the course of the disease.[11] Servimed also offers an experimental treatment for vitiligo, a skin pigmentation disorder, using human placenta tissue, as well as addition therapies and more conventional health services. The Cuban state enterprise also advertises cosmetic surgeries, although the International Society of Aesthetic Plastic Surgery, which promotes safety in world health tourism, does not list any Cuban surgeons or clinics among its accredited facilities in thirty-six countries.[12]

Other Cuban health care professionals may simply choose to emigrate, despite the uncertainty of passing the licensing requirements in other countries and finding jobs in the field. Many Cuban doctors have already abandoned the profession to seek work in the tourist sector, and anecdotal accounts of physicians working in hotels and as taxi drivers abound. In order to maintain the public health system, salaries will have to be boosted considerably. A number of Cuban physicians already treat patients privately, charging under-the-table fees. In 2012, Cuban police interrogated an undisclosed number of doctors and other health personnel from two Havana hospitals accused of performing surgeries on paying patients at public hospitals and using private residences as recovery rooms.[13]

Meanwhile, the provision of primary health care has deteriorated. There were 61 million medical consultations in 2013, including 41 million at the primary care level in 2013, according to Cuban Health Minister Dr. Roberto Morales Ojeda, who presented a report to the Council of State.[14] But these figures, if accurate, represented a significant decline from the previous year: according to figures published by Cuba's national statistics office, there were over 66 million primary care consultations in 2012, out of more than 81 million medical visits overall.[15] There are credible and detailed accounts from Cubans themselves of family doctor-and-nurse *consultorios* closed or abandoned by health personnel, without explanation.[16] A brief report in Cuba's weekly labor newspaper *Trabajadores* said that over 100,000 jobs in the health care sector had been cut, but offered no details.[17] The government had earlier announced a pay hike for its medical personnel, with top-ranked physicians receiving salary increases from 627 pesos to 1,600 pesos, or about US$61 per month. Nurses' salaries would be raised from 320 to 595 pesos, or $22 per month.[18]

During the authors' consultations with Cuban doctors who had left the country, we usually posed the following hypothetical question: Imagine that a transition government is in place. You have been invited to take part on a panel that will make recommendations for improving health care in the future. What might your recommendations be?

One doctor pointed out that Cuban official secrecy made it impossible to know what resources were available and the true extent of the country's health needs. All wanted Cuba to continue to have a public health system available to everyone, but said that doctors should also be allowed to practice privately. One possibility might be to allow physicians working in the public health system to work part-time in private practice, as do many in Britain's National Health Service and other countries. Darsi Ferrer, a physician and former political prisoner whose case was supported by Amnesty International, said that health tourism might continue, but that the profits should be reinvested in Cuba's public health system.[19]

Many Cuba specialists predict that the country is unlikely to undergo any major political transformation immediately after the Castro brothers leave the scene, as there are several of their close collaborators waiting in the wings, who control various state enterprises and who would have much to lose in the event of systemic change. A full normalization of U.S.–Cuba relations also seems unlikely for the time being, though existing restrictions on travel and trade might be further loosened.

Even so, a different Cuban leader might be willing to allow more NGOs to work in the country, which would open the way for more donations of medical supplies and other humanitarian assistance. Such assistance, at least initially, seems likely to run into bureaucratic obstacles and logistical problems of the sort experienced by Canadian groups described in chapter 2, and may be confronted with a nationalistic backlash on the part some sectors of Cuban officialdom. In 2012 a Florida shipping company was authorized to transport humanitarian donations to Cuba but the service ended less than a year later due to financial problems and infrastructure bottlenecks. Cuban customs officials, who use paper records rather than computers to track shipments, could not keep up with the sheer volume of packages Florida residents were sending to family and friends, and what was supposed to be a weekly shipping service was reduced to a monthly shipment before finally halting altogether.[20]

The activities of NGOs require coordination in order to be effective, and without coordination some groups may embark on individual projects with a short-term focus. NGOs will have to take care not to engage in activities which might draw patients away from existing health facilities and instead direct their efforts toward supporting the abilities of primary care providers to treat their patients.

Some opportunities for NGOs might lie in helping maintain the country's blood banks and vaccination programs, as well as support projects to help Cubans with HIV/AIDS and other infectious diseases. One significant area of need will be the collection and coordination of epidemiological data between NGOs and Cuban state health authorities.

There is also the possibility of more cooperation in the field of medical research between the two countries, building on some of the relationships already in place. Atlanta's Center for Disease Control has worked with Cuba's Health Tendencies Analysis Unit, founded during the 1992–1993 epidemic of optic and peripheral neuropathy. According to director Dr. Daniel Rodriguez Milord, this collaboration involved "looking at how they designed their surveillance system and analyzing how to design and improve ours."[21] Harvard University and the Pedro Kouri Institute for Tropical Medicine also have a longstanding relationship that includes joint research projects into HIV/AIDS, tuberculosis, dengue fever, and a variety of other illnesses.[22]

Cuba's biotechnology sector has been weakened by a lack of funding and in the words of Dr. Cesar Reynel, who worked in the field in the early 1990s, "scientific practices contaminated by political orientation."[23] While the country has more than its share of well-trained and capable professionals, the sector's profitability will drop if it has to start paying scientists decent salaries, he said.

According to Dr. Jose de la Fuente, who also worked in the industry during its early stages, the sector might be revived with more investment and the ability of its scientists to freely interact with their colleagues at the international level. At present, Cuban scientists' access to overseas meetings and conferences in their fields is granted on the basis of political reliability as much as professional accomplishments. There is also the possibility of forming joint ventures with U.S. or European groups, he said [24]

When U.S.–Cuban relations are normalized, the island may become an attractive retirement destination for older Americans, especially Cuban-Americans. While Medicare benefits are not extended to U.S. citizens residing overseas, there are significant cost-saving potential benefits to consider. The price of hip replacement surgery in an internationally accredited hospital in Costa Rica, another destination for American retirees, is often less than half of what it is in the United States and a number of countries offer foreign residents comprehensive health coverage plans for a fraction of the cost of U.S. health insurance coverage.[25]

Should the 1965 Social Security Act be amended to allow payments to health care providers outside the United States, Cuban hospitals and clinics that already serve foreign tourists would enjoy additional revenues (which hopefully would be shared with the country's public health system), provided they meet certain international standards of care. One first step might be for one of the Miami-based Health Management Organizations (HMOs) with Cuban-American personnel and clientele to expand operations to Havana. If successful, this plan might lead to a revival of the mutualist health associations which once provided reasonably priced medical services to roughly half of Havana's population, as described in chapter 1. In the best of all cases, American HMOs, the Cuban mutualist health associations and Cuba's public health sector could play complementary roles, with the first two helping to relieve the pressure on the third sector.[26]

The Latin American Medical School will probably continue its intake of paying students under bilateral agreements with other developing countries. But in order for such accords to remain viable, more efforts will be needed to bridge the gap between the foreign students' medical education in Cuba and the requirements for practicing the profession in their own countries. This will inevitably mean improving relations with the professional medical societies in other countries, which have not always been receptive to the presence of Cuban doctors and have raised questions about the cost and quality of Cuban medical training.

The United States has a shortage of primary care doctors, which if current trends continue could reach 45,000 unfilled posts by 2020, according to the Association of American Medical Colleges (AAMC), as well as a deficit of 46,000 specialists, "leaving patients with cancer, Alzheimer's disease and dementia, hip fractures, and other ailments without immediate access to care."[27] If the Latin American School of Medicine were able to work with U.S. medical educators in developing a program for American students, then Cuba could help fill this need. U.S. graduates of some foreign medical programs have a high pass rate when taking the United States Medical Licensing Exam (USMLE); St. George's University Medical School in Grenada boasts a 97 percent pass rate for its American students.[28]

Another possibility might be for Cuba to expand the training of nurses, a profession for which there is a critical shortage in both developing and industrialized countries. Having adequate numbers of nurses on staff has been linked to improved patient outcomes at hospitals, including a shortening of patients' length of stay as well as a reduction in adverse outcomes such as urinary tract infections, gastrointestinal bleeding, hospital-acquired pneumonia, shock, and cardiac arrest.[29] The United States' shortage of nurses has been estimated at 135,000, and one survey revealed that 55 percent of nurses working in the country planned to retire between 2011 and 2020, and the number of those entering the profession is less than those leaving.[30] Providing nursing services to other countries also offers a potential source of revenue for Cuba.

As discussed in the last chapter, Cuba's medical assistance programs abroad have given way to contracted medical services with governments in Brazil and other countries and these agreements seem likely to grow in the near future. This may cause more depletion of medical staff in Cuba, and the country's economic constraints mitigate against many overseas humanitarian programs in the future, except in cases where other countries or international agencies help fund the projects. The future focus will necessarily be on providing care to the Cuban people and finding ways to pay for it. But Cuban doctors, working in far-flung areas around the world, have earned themselves considerable goodwill. And given its long medical tradition—a tradition which began centuries before the Castro government—it seems certain that Cuba will always have its medical heroes.

NOTES

1. "Vivienda en Cuba: el derrumbe que viene," *Cafe Fuerte*, July 8, 2013,
2. Dinorah de la Caridad Oliva Venereo, Clarivel Saavedra Ramírez, Arturo Luis Viñas Martínez; Caridad de la Torre Silva, "Características epidemiológicas del VIH/SIDA en las mujeres de Ciudad de La Habana," *Revista Cubana de Medicina* Vol. 49, No. 1 (2010), pp. 1–6.
3. Ibid.
4. Mario Hechavarría Driggs, "Cuba: Hepatitis A en un municipio habanero y alerta por cólera en Villa Clara," *El Correo de Cuba*, March 28, 2014, http://www.elcorreodecuba.com/cuba/noticias/604-cuba-hepatitis-a-en-municipio-habanero-y-alerta-por-colera-villa-clara
5. "Cuba Cancer Patients Suffer from Health Care Negligence," *Havana Times*, January 9, 2014, http://www.havanatimes.org/?p=101124
6. Laurie Garrett, "Castrocare in Crisis: Will Lifting the Embargo Make Things Worse?" *Foreign Affairs*, July/August 2010.
7. P. Sean Brotherton, *Revolutionary Medicine: Health and the Body in Post-Soviet Cuba* (Durham, NC: Duke University Press, 2012), p. 161.
8. Ibid, p. 159.
9. Dr. Hilda Molina, "Cuban Medicine Today," http://www.futurodecuba.org/ARticle%20by%20Dra_%20Molina.htm.
10. "Programa Cubana por el tratamiento de Retinitis Pigmentosa," http://www.servimedcuba.com/index.php?option=com_content&view=article&id=102&Itemid=223.
11. Institut Nazareth e Louis Braille, "Is there evidence supporting the Cuban treatment for retinitis pigmentosa?" http://www.inlb.qc.ca/librairies/sfv/telecharger.php?fichier=1232.
12. "ISAPS Accredited Facilities by Country," http://www.isaps.org/find-a-surgeon/accredited/.
13. Juan O. Tamayo, "Cuban doctors treated private patients in public hospitals," *Miami Herald*, July 20, 2012.
14. *Granma*, December 23, 2013.
15. Anuario Estadistico de Salud 2012, http://files.sld.cu/dne/files/2013/04/anuario_2012.pdf.
16. See for example, "El médico de cabecera no está, señor," *Cubanet*, January 7, 2014, http://www.cubanet.org/articulos/el-medico-de-cabecera-no-esta-senor/, in which the author toured primary care facilities in four Havana municipalities and found nine closed, without explanation. The sign outside one of the doctor's offices said it cared for 1,354 patients—a considerably higher number than the official doctor-to-patient numbers cited by Cuban officials.
17. "Cuba Slashes more than 100,000 Health Care Jobs," *Associated Press*, April 7, 2014.

18. Juan O. Tamayo, "Cuba hikes pay for doctors at home and abroad." *Miami Herald*, March 21, 2014.
19. Interview with Darsi Ferrer, April 18, 2013.
20. Christine Armario, "Shipping to Cuba from Miami by Sea Stops After International Port Corp's Big Start," *Associated Press*, April 8, 2013.
21. Connor Gorry, "Training and Eye on Epidemics: Cuba's National Health Surveillance System." *MEDICC Review*, Vol. 7, No. 7 (July 2005), http://www.medicc.org/publications/medicc_review/0705/mr-features.html.
22. Harvard University David Rockefeller Center for Latin American Studies, "Faculty Research and Initiatives on Cuba," http://drclas.harvard.edu/pages/faculty-research-and-initiatives-cuba.
23. Interview with Dr. Cesar Reynel, October 16, 2013.
24. Interview with Dr. Jose de la Fuente, November 12, 2013.
25. Stacy Julien, "If I Go Abroad, What Happens to My Medicare?" AARP blog, posted August 22, 2012, http://blog.aarp.org/2012/08/22/if-i-go-abroad-what-happens-to-my-medicare/.
26. Sergio Diaz-Briquets, "Medicare: A Potential Income-Generating Activity for Cuba in the Future," Cuba in Transition, Association for the Study of the Cuban Economy, 2001.
27. "Washington Highlights: Senate Panel Discusses Primary Care Shortages," Association of American Medical Colleges, February 1, 2013, https://www.aamc.org/advocacy/washhigh/highlights2013/327196/020113senatepaneldiscussesprimarycareshortages.html#.Us8MutI7uSp.
28. According to its website, St George's University students taking the USMLE for the first time achieved a 97 percent pass rate. http://www.sgu.edu/future-students/faqs.html
29. J. Needleman, P. Buerhous, S. Mattke, M. Stewart, and K. Zelevinsky, "Nurse–Staffing Levels and Quality of Care in Hospitals," *New England Journal of Medicine* Vol. 336, No. 22.
30. Robert Rosseter, "Nursing Shortage," AACN, May 3, 2010. http://www.aacn.nche.edu/media-relations/fact-sheets/nursing-shortage. Accessed January 28, 2010.

Appendix 1: Cuban Doctors' Open Letter to Raul Castro, Which Began Circulating in September 2012

Open letter from the General Surgery Department of the "Calixto Garcia" Hospital to the First Secretary of the Cuban Communist Party and President of the Councils of State and Ministers, Army General Raul Castro Ruz

> To be good is the only way to be happy. To be cultured is the only way to be free. But, given human nature, one needs to be prosperous to be good. —José Martí

The "Calixto Garcia" hospital in Havana takes as its mission to provide specialized preventative-curative medical care and rehabilitation without interruption to the population through high-quality medical care and high professional standards [1]. With its 100-year history it has been a permanent school of surgeons in the country, and an important element in our country's struggle for independence; many of our professors were clandestine combatants [2] and brilliant doctors on international medical missions of great importance. Surgeons at the hospital, respecting the Hippocratic Oath [3], have historically been characterized as being critical and self-critical, but especially combative in the face of difficulties, bad decisions taken, and the multiple errors that affect our nation, and that little by little are endangering the future, taking health as a pillar of the transformations arising in the Revolutionary period, and our duty to provide a professional and dignified medical care, in accord with the scientific advances of the 21st century.

After countless reports to the head of the service, hospital management, discussions within the core of the Cuban Communist Party, and our long standing inability to participate in discussion at other levels with the leaders of the ministry, where medical personnel present their uncensored opinions [8] and ways to solve the major problems currently plaguing the health sector, which include everything from training to direct care, a group of surgeons felt it their elementary duty [8, 9, 10] and agreed to send this letter to the head of the service, for the sole purpose of informing him of the extremely serious elements in healthcare delivery to the Cuban people, which apparently at this time when it is happening in public health in general, and in our hospital in particular, the lack of immediate plans to resolve them are unknown by the top political leadership of the country, contrasting inversely with the official discourse of our media.

Medical care, and especially surgery in our center is a great disaster, characterized by:

- A hospital with a destroyed physical structure, due to its age and innumerable poor quality and short-term repairs.
- A lack of important resources for the care of patients, because of inadequate distribution, insufficient management, or excess work because of the reduction of this activity in other hospitals for similar reasons.
- Human mental deterioration accompanied by the loss of the minimum attention to the person, who spends long days of free labor for a significant number of hours, and in a country where the "free perks" have been ended, and where working conditions are below those of any poor place in the world.

In our hospital the surgical services have been declining and the number of operating rooms has been reduced from about 30 for all specialties to no more than 10 at present, which although greatly destroyed still provide this vital service to the people. The irregularities in these operating rooms, their constantly broken air conditioning, lack of water, lack of adequate equipment in some of them, means that cancer patients cannot be operated on in time in our institution, others with benign conditions, susceptible to immediate treatment when diagnosed, develop complications because of delays in the resolution of their problems.

And as if that weren't enough, the urgent conditions also present great difficulties. These, which constitute an important number of cases, are referred from some other place in the city, many times transferred poorly, which puts the lives of these patients in danger and even kills them when theoretically this could have been avoided. Despite the fact this this is the only surgical priority this hospital serves a good part of the time, they must sometimes wait more than 24 hours between their arrival and their emergency surgery, mainly because of the lack of available operating rooms and of sufficient and adequate personnel, but also because of the physical exhaustion of the doctors who raise these issues and raise them again and discuss these problems at every possible level and/or a good part of the time put the responsibility on the orderlies, cleaners, and in addition put the full responsibility for sick patients on their families, the sick patients themselves, and society.

The deficiencies in the health care system are so serious, in our opinion, that we are forced by these issues and others of resources that continue in a temporary or permanent way, to provide care to our people that is not professionally ethical or dignified, as is our sacred duty.

Moreover, the repairs undertaken at our hospital, that have been underway for more than 10 years, have done little to change the unviability of a horizontal hospital in current times; the majority of the repairs are putting make-up on old buildings, performed with terrible quality and, of course, lasting a short time, which increases the frequency of new repairs.

Rooms that have waited 10 years for repairs, today crumble four months after they open, with the first downpour; leaks, collapses of the false ceilings, and a number of important areas declared inhabitable, are a daily fact of life in our work and our patients' stays.

The suspension of operations because of the weather, water, insufficient rooms, or whatever cause, is no longer unforeseen but rather is commonplace. As the operating rooms are no longer available to solve the problems of the patients, now it is us, the surgeons, who must prioritize one or another patient in an an unfortunate and exhausting search for surgical opportunities for a Cuban whom we only know, sadly, because of his illness.

The only thing we need to add to this depressing picture is the working conditions of the doctors and the personnel in general, starting with wages that are not enough to support a family, degrading working conditions; including lack of a place to rest during long days of surgery or work, the several miles walked between rooms, in the dust, the sun, and many times the rain; the terrible quality and quantity of food; the lack of a decent place to take care of one's physiological needs; and no showers to cool off in the intense heat or to clean up before contaminating a surgery, almost force us, when they become permanent, to change our mentality.

The fatigue leads to well studied complications [4, 5, 6, 7]; if on top of that we add the ridiculous figure of 2-1/2 gallons of gas a month for those fortunate enough to have cars, not even enough to go to and from work for the first week of the month, among many other mistreatments; it all completes the picture of deteriorations that definitely have a bearing on the medical care that is offered to the people.

Today it is impossible to ask doctors, even with a car, to come to the hospital in the middle of the night to check on their surgical patients, or to come on Sunday, as was common among surgeons historically; and what's more it's impossible to ask them to perform a new operation on a patient with complications at 10 PM and you don't have to be very intelligent to know what happens with a case when a patient has been repeatedly operated on five times by different surgeons.

We believe that this situation generates unquestionably disastrous complications in patients, where studies show that after six hours of work of a surgeon's complications multiply [4, 5, 6, 7]; and of course, that's talking about working with appropriate comfort. Also in many cases, death, which we cause when we have a terminal patient with almost no hope; it is not ethically dignified because we can't do for him what he deserves or should have, at the time it should be done: we have multiple examples from all the surgeons who work in this hospital, and the great number of the population who observe and criticize, that what is said in the media has no connection to our country and our hospitals.

We think that our government has a commitment in all this, because it exists to meet the needs of the people, to solve the problems of the people, of the workers, simply because they are responsible for maintaining the hospitals, for properly training the workers in a high quality and fair educational system, for developing an ethical education consistent with the work they will be doing, or anyone thinks why do doctors, engineers, builders undertake the missions they do in their work: they do it because their work makes things better, for their family and the society they live in, but unfortunately that is only achieved in our country by leaving it, leaving the country that gave us birth [10], which is ours by right, and nobody, absolutely nobody, has the right to take away our identity under any circumstances, and for which we must give even our lives for our nation to remain independent.

The misfortunes narrated here do not come alone, they come about slowly when the investment is maintained for years in the living standards of the people with their ability and dedications, the socialist law well known by everyone: "to everyone according to his work." When the leaders, with their laws, decrees, special circulars, and their decisions and provisions, are compromising the future, how long will we thank the centenary generation for having fulfilled their duty and obligation of liberating Cuba, while our generation wants to fulfill its duty to develop and give our families, our children, our Cuban brothers, the life they deserve, while the destructive tracks of corruption run riot with a singular debauchery on every side of society where we turn our gaze?

As José Martí said: "given human nature, one needs to be prosperous to be good." The government is responsible for all this, not only for knowing it, but also for fixing it. So, and before it's too late, leading to events like those at the Mazorra hospital [where 40+ patients starved and froze to death], we decided in this group of doctors, sacrificing, hardworking, dedicated, ethical, and above all badly treated, to report to you and to those responsible all of our concerns, in our modest opinion serious ones, from this place so undervalued on the social scale, which is the heroic and historical general surgery service of the oldest hospital in our beloved country.

Notes:

[1] http://bvs.sld.cu/cgi-bin/wxis/dis1/

[2] http://files.sld.cu/cirured/files/2011/06/de-mis-memorias.pdf

[3] Juramento Hipocrático. www.sld.cu

[4] Editorial. Revista Canadian Medical Association Journal http://www.cmaj.ca/

[5] Journal of the American Medical Association

[6] http://www.elmundo.es/elmundosalud/2011/05/24/noticias/1306246063.html

[7] http://www.elmundo.es/blogs/salud/profesionsanitaria/2011/05/18/un-tacografo-para-los-medicos.html

[8] "Now whomever wants to speak will speak, good or bad, but whoever wants to will speak. Not as happened here, when only those who spoke evil spoke, there will be freedom." Speech by Fidel Castro. Parque Cespedes, Santiago de Cuba, on January 1, 1959.

[9] ". . . How can we say 'this is our homeland' if the homeland does not have anything? 'My homeland', but my homeland does not give me anything, my homeland does not sustain me, in my homeland I'm starving. That's not a homeland! Will the homeland be for a few, but not a homeland for the people. Homeland does not mean only a place where one can shout, talk and walk without being killed; homeland is a place where you can live, homeland is a place where you can work and earn an honest living, and also earn what is fair pay for your work. Homeland is where the citizen is not exploited, because if they exploit the citizen, if you take away what belongs to him, if you steal what he has, that is not homeland." Speech by Fidel Castro Ruz, at the Town Square of Camagüey, on January 4, 1959.

[10] ". . . it is precisely the tragedy of our people not to have a homeland. And the best evidence, the best evidence that we have no homeland is that tens of thousands of children of this land are leaving Cuba for another country to live, but they have no homeland. And not everyone who wants to leave goes, only those who can. And that's true and you know it." Speech by Fidel Castro Ruz, at the Town Square of Camagüey, on January 4, 1959.

Appendix 2: A Cuban Medical Timeline

1728 Cuba's first medical school is established with the founding of the University of Havana.

1795 Dr. Tomas Romay publishes an article on smallpox vaccination.

1835 Central Vaccine Board founded.

1852 El Criterio, Cuba's first medical journal appears.

1881 Cuban physician Carlos Finlay becomes the first to theorize that yellow fever is carried by a mosquito.

1937 The Institute for Tropical Medicine is founded at the University of Havana.

1959 The rebel army led by Fidel Castro seizes control of Cuba.

1960 The first Cuban overseas medical mission is sent to Chile following an earthquake.

1962 Cuba begins a nationwide vaccination campaign.

1963 The Cuban Ministry of Health and Welfare is renamed the Ministry of Public Health and charged with administering all medical services in the country.

1967 The Castro government takes over the last of the mutualist clinics.

1981 Cuba suffers an outbreak of dengue fever, affecting 344,203 people. In a speech Fidel Castro says he suspects the United States is behind the epidemic.

1984 Cuba begins the family doctor program, with the stated goal of placing a doctor-nurse team in every neighborhood in the country.

1985 The first AIDS case is diagnosed in Cuba, a heterosexual man returning from an international mission.

1986 Cuba's first death from AIDS is announced; the government begins a controversial program to place HIV/AIDS patients in quarantined sanatoria.

1997 Cuba experiences another outbreak of dengue fever, beginning in the eastern part of the country. Dessy Mendoza, a Cuban doctor who reported the epidemic, is arrested and sentenced to eight years imprisonment for "spreading enemy propaganda."

2006 Cuba signs an "oil for doctors" accord with Venezuela.

2010 The Cuban government announces that foreign visitors must have health insurance.

2011 Venezuelan president Hugo Chavez undergoes cancer surgery in Cuba, and continues to receive treatment in Cuba for his undisclosed type of cancer for nearly two years, flying back and forth between Caracas and Havana.

2013 Cuba and Brazil sign an agreement in which Cuba will provide doctors to work in underserved areas.

2014 The Cuban government announces pay hikes for medical personnel, and reveals it has cut over 100,000 health care jobs over the past two years.

Selected Bibliography

Books

Brotherton, P. Sean. *Revolutionary Medicine: Health and the Body in Post-Soviet Cuba.* Durham, NC: Duke University Press, 2012.

Danielson, Ross. *Cuban Medicine.* New Brunswick, NJ: Transaction Books, 1979.

Diaz-Briquets, Sergio. *The Health Revolution in Cuba.* Austin, University of Texas Press, 1983.

Diaz-Briquets, Sergio and Jorge Perez-Lopez. *Corruption in Cuba: Castro and Beyond.* Austin: University of Texas Press, 2006.

Feinsilver, Julie. *Healing the Masses: Cuban Health Politics at Home and Abroad.* Berkeley: University of California Press, 1993.

Garfield, Richard and Timothy Holtz, eds. *Health System reforms in Cuba in the 1990s.* London: Institute of Latin American Studies, 2000.

Hirschfeld, Katherine, *Health, Politics and Revolution in Cuba Since 1898.* New Brunswick, NJ: Transaction Publishers, 2009.

MacDonald, Theodore H. *A Developmental Analysis of Cuba's Health Care System Since 1959.* Queenston, UK: The Edwin Mellen Press, 1999.

Macintyre, K., and J. Hadad. "Cuba," in *World Health Systems Challenges and Perspectives,* eds. B. Fried and L. Gaydos. Chicago: Health Administration Press, 2002.

Reports

American Association for World Health, "Denial of Food and Medicine: The Impact of the U.S. Embargo on Health and Nutrition in Cuba," March 1997.

De Gordon, A. M. "Health and Health Care in Cuba: The Transition from Socialism to the Future." Unpublished manuscript, 2003.

Garcia-Quinones, Rolando. "Social policies, family arrangements and population aging in Cuba." United Nations Population Fund, June 2009.

Hernandez Castellon, Rafael, "Population Ageing in Cuba," Center for Demographic Studies, University of Havana, 1994.

Organization of American States (OAS). "Situation of Human Rights in Cuba." Inter-American Commission on Human Rights, 1983. Retrieved April 1, 2003, from http://www.cidh.oas.org/countryrep/Cuba83eng/chap.13.htm.

Oxfam America and Washington Office on Latin America (WOLA). "Myths and Facts about the U.S. Embargo on Medicine and Medical Supplies." Washington, D.C., 1997.

Pan American Health Organization (PAHO). "Health in the Americas: Cuba." Washington D.C.: United Nations Publications: 206-219. 1998.

———. "Cuba. Profile of the Health Services System." Washington D.C.: Division of Health Systems and Services Develipment: 1-23. 1999.

Sixto, Felipe ."An Evaluation of Four Decades of Cuban Healthcare: Cuba in Transition." Association for the Study of the Cuban Economy, 2002.

Werlau, Maria C. "Cuba-Venezuela Health Diplomacy: The Politics of Humanitarianism." Cuba in Transition, Association for the Study for the Study of the Cuban Economy, 2010.

———. "Cuba's Business of Humanitarianism: The Medical Mission in Haiti." Cuba in Transition, Association for the Study of the Cuban Economy, 2011.

———. "The Effects of the U.S. Embargo on Health and Nutrition in Cuba: A Critical Analysis." Cuba in Transition. Association for the Study of the Cuban Economy, 1998.

Index

About the Authors

Mary Helen Spooner is a journalist who has covered Latin American topics since 1977. She is the author of *Soldiers in a Narrow Land: The Pinochet Regime in Chile* (1999) and *The General's Slow Retreat: Chile after Pinochet* (2011). She blogs at notesontheamericas.wordpress.com.

Dr. Steven Ullmann is director of the Center for Programs in Health Sector Management and Policy at the University of Miami. He is professor in the Department of Management and holds secondary appointments in the Department of Economics in the School of Business, and in the Departments of Epidemiology and Public Health, and Family Medicine and Community Health in the Miller School of Medicine. He specializes in the areas of health care management, health care economics, and medical ethics. His research has focused on quality and efficiency of health care, health care for an aging population, the impact of health technology on quality and costs, and the linkages between environment and health care costs and outcomes. Dr. Ullmann's work has taken him to countries in Asia, Europe, Latin America, and the Caribbean.

www.ingramcontent.com/pod-product-compliance
Lightning Source LLC
Chambersburg PA
CBHW031414220926
51612CB00004B/4
* 9 7 8 0 7 3 9 1 7 6 0 3 0 *